Bovine Clinical Pharmacology

Editor

MICHAEL D. APLEY

VETERINARY CLINICS OF NORTH AMERICA: FOOD ANIMAL PRACTICE

www.vetfood.theclinics.com

Consulting Editor
ROBERT A. SMITH

March 2015 • Volume 31 • Number 1

ELSEVIER

1600 John F. Kennedy Boulevard • Suite 1800 • Philadelphia, Pennsylvania, 19103-2899

http://www.vetfood.theclinics.com

VETERINARY CLINICS OF NORTH AMERICA: FOOD ANIMAL PRACTICE Volume 31, Number 1
March 2015 ISSN 0749-0720, ISBN-13: 978-0-323-35668-8

Editor: Patrick Manley
Developmental Editor: Meredith Clinton

Veterinary Clinics of North America: Food Animal Practice (ISSN 0749-0720) is published in March, July, and November by Elsevier Inc., 360 Park Avenue South, New York, NY 10010-1710. Subscription prices are $235.00 per year (domestic individuals), $326.00 per year (domestic institutions), $110.00 per year (domestic students/residents), $265.00 per year (Canadian individuals), $430.00 per year (Canadian institutions), $335.00 per year (international individuals), $430.00 per year (international institutions), and $165.00 per year (international and Canadian students/residents). To receive student/resident rate, orders must be accompanied by name of affiliated institution, date of term, and the signature of program/residency coordinator on institution letterhead. *Clinics* subscription prices. All prices are subject to change without notice. **POSTMASTER:** Send address changes to *Veterinary Clinics of North America: Food Animal Practice*, Elsevier Health Sciences Division, Subscription Customer Service, 3251 Riverport Lane, Maryland Heights, MO 63043. Customer Service (orders, claims, online, change of address): Elsevier Health Sciences Division, Subscription Customer Service, 3251 Riverport Lane, Maryland Heights, MO 63043. Tel: 1-800-654-2452 (U.S. and Canada); 314-447-8871 (ouside U.S. and Canada). Fax: 314-447-8029. E-mail: journalscustomerservice-usa@elsevier.com (for print support); journalsonlinesupport-usa@elsevier.com (for online support).

Reprints. For copies of 100 or more, of articles in this publication, please contact the Commercial Reprints Department, Elsevier Inc., 360 Park Avenue South, New York, NY 10010-1710. Tel.: 212-633-3874; Fax: 212-633-3820; E-mail: reprints@elsevier.com.

Veterinary Clinics of North America: Food Animal Practice is covered in *Current Contents/Agriculture, Biology and Environmental Sciences, MEDLINE/PubMed (Index Medicus), and Excerpta Medica.*

Contributors

CONSULTING EDITOR

ROBERT A. SMITH, DVM, MS
Diplomate, American Board of Veterinary Practitioners; Veterinary Research and Consulting Services, LLC, Greeley, Colorado

EDITOR

MICHAEL D. APLEY, DVM, PhD
Diplomate, American College of Veterinary Clinical Pharmacology; Professor, Department of Clinical Sciences, Kansas State University College of Veterinary Medicine, Manhattan, Kansas

AUTHORS

JOHN A. ANGELOS, MS, DVM, PhD
Diplomate, American College of Veterinary Internal Medicine; Associate Professor, Department of Medicine and Epidemiology, University of California, Davis, California

MICHAEL D. APLEY, DVM, PhD
Diplomate, American College of Veterinary Clinical Pharmacology; Professor, Department of Clinical Sciences, Kansas State University College of Veterinary Medicine, Manhattan, Kansas

JOHANN F. COETZEE, BVSc, Cert CHP, PhD, MRCVS
Diplomate, American College of Veterinary Clinical Pharmacology; Diplomate, American College of Animal Welfare; Professor, Department of Veterinary Diagnostic and Production Animal Medicine, College of Veterinary Medicine, Iowa State University, Ames, Iowa

KEITH D. DeDONDER, MS, DVM
Department of Diagnostic Medicine/Pathobiology, Kansas State University College of Veterinary Medicine, Manhattan, Kansas

VIRGINIA FAJT, DVM, PhD
Diplomate, American College of Veterinary Clinical Pharmacology; Clinical Associate Professor, Veterinary Physiology and Pharmacology, Texas A&M University College of Veterinary Medicine and Biomedical Sciences, College Station, Texas

BRIAN LUBBERS, DVM, PhD
Diplomate, American College of Veterinary Clinical Pharmacology; Director, Clinical Microbiology, Kansas State Veterinary Diagnostic Laboratory, Kansas State University, Manhattan, Kansas

ANNETTE O'CONNOR, MVSc, DVSc, FANZCVSc
Professor of Epidemiology, Veterinary Medical Research Institute, College of Veterinary Medicine, Iowa State University, Ames, Iowa

EMILY J. REPPERT, DVM, MS
Assistant Professor Food Animal, Department of Clinical Sciences, Veterinary Health Center, Kansas State University, Manhattan, Kansas

ERIN ROYSTER, DVM, MS
Instructor in Dairy Production Medicine, Department of Veterinary Population Medicine, College of Veterinary Medicine, University of Minnesota, Saint Paul, Minnesota

GEOF SMITH, DVM, MS, PhD
Diplomate, American College of Veterinary Internal Medicine; Professor, Department of Population Health & Pathobiology, North Carolina State University, Raleigh, North Carolina

MATTHEW L. STOCK, VMD
Diplomate, American Board of Veterinary Practitioners (Food Animal Practice); Graduate Assistant, Department of Veterinary Diagnostic and Production Animal Medicine, College of Veterinary Medicine, Iowa State University, Ames, Iowa

SARAH WAGNER, DVM, PhD
Diplomate, American College of Veterinary Clinical Pharmacology; Associate Professor, Department of Animal Sciences, North Dakota State University, Fargo, North Dakota

Contents

include consideration of the host, the environment, herd management, and ongoing surveillance even after the immediate crisis has passed. Research over many years has led to the discovery of a variety of antibiotic treatments and antibiotic regimens that can be effective against IBK. The discoveries of Mor bovoculi and reports of IBK associated with Mycoplasma spp without concurrent Mor bovis or Mor bovoculi have raised new questions into the roles that other organisms may play in IBK pathogenesis.

Data supporting individual animal therapy for papillomatous digital dermatitis (PDD) and infectious pododermatitis (IP) in cattle are available for treatment with multiple drugs in the form of randomized, prospective clinical trials conducted in naturally occurring disease with negative controls and masked subjective evaluators. In the case of PDD, these trials support the use of topical tetracycline and oxytetracycline, lincomycin, a copper-containing preparation, and a nonantimicrobial cream. In individual therapy for IP, trial evidence is available to support systemic treatment with ceftiofur, florfenicol, tulathromycin, and oxytetracycline. However, it was not available for IP standards such as penicillin G, sulfadimethoxine, and tylosin.

Bovine respiratory disease (BRD) remains a major disease from an economic and an animal welfare standpoint in beef production systems. Antimicrobial administration is a mainstay in the control of and therapeutic treatment of acute BRD. Judicious use of antimicrobials remains paramount to ensure efficacy of treatment remains acceptable. A systemic review was conducted in the scientific literature, the objective of which was to present a cumulative review of the data from published randomized clinical trials using a negative control in the treatment and control of BRD and using the number needed to treat as a means to effectively convey this information to bovine practitioners.

Providing pain relief in cattle is challenging. In the absence of labeled drugs, the Animal Medicinal Drug Use Clarification Act regulates the extralabel drug use of analgesics in cattle within the United States. Given the variety of pharmacokinetic and pharmacodynamic properties of pain-relieving drugs, evidence needs to drive the development of analgesic protocols for cattle during pain-related events. This article reviews the commonly used analgesics investigated in cattle including local anesthetics, nonsteroidal anti-inflammatory drugs, opioids, α2-agonists, N-methyl-D-aspartate receptor antagonists, and gabapentin. These compounds are examined with respect to evidence of analgesia in cattle during pain states.

Metritis is a cause of postparturient uterine disease in dairy cattle and is most commonly associated with watery fetid red-brown uterine discharge occurring in the first 21 days postpartum. The most severe form of metritis (puerperal metritis) often warrants antibiotic therapy. This article analyzes the current literature to determine the efficacy of ceftiofur in the treatment of metritis. Evidence-based review of the current literature suggests that there is evidence for the use of ceftiofur in the treatment of metritis. However, review of the literature also reveals the need for more studies with negative control groups.

Randomized, masked, prospective clinical trial evidence for therapeutic intervention in naturally occurring bovine polioencephalomalacia (polio) is nonexistent. This article evaluates the use of thiamine and anti-inflammatories in the therapy of polioencephalomalacia based on available information related to the pathophysiology of the disease, induced models, disease outcome in other species (sheep), and parallels in similar disease in humans.

The integration of antimicrobial susceptibility test results into food animal case management can be a challenging proposition. The use of Clinical and Laboratory Standards Institute veterinary-specific interpretive criteria can assist with the antimicrobial selection process when these criteria exist for the specific antimicrobial, pathogen, host animal, disease process, and dosing regimen being considered. When veterinary-specific interpretive criteria do not exist, clinicians can, and should, evaluate microbiological, pharmacological and clinical data to ensure responsible use of antimicrobials.

VETERINARY CLINICS OF NORTH AMERICA: FOOD ANIMAL PRACTICE

Preface

Making Clinical Decisions in Cases with and without the Support of Clinical Trials

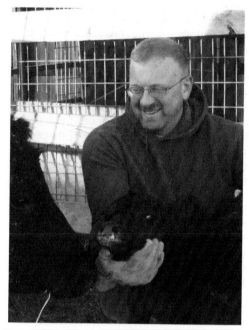

Michael D. Apley, DVM, PhD, DACVCP
Editor

The practice of food animal veterinary medicine continues to evolve, and much of this evolution is based on data gathering and analysis. We now have more prospective, controlled, randomized, masked clinical trials to guide us in major diseases such as bovine respiratory disease and mastitis. For these diseases, our task becomes critical appraisal of the available data and how the results may or may not apply to a specific clinical situation (ie, the external relevance of the studies). On the other end of the spectrum, such as for polioencephalomalacia, we are left to evaluate physiologic reasoning along with induced models and clinical trials in other species, and possibly other diseases, for guidance.

As food animal veterinarians, preventive programs are a priority pursuing our primary goal of avoiding the need for therapeutic intervention in disease. But when disease is present, we must intervene. To sit idly by in a fit of indecision due to a lack of

Vet Clin Food Anim 31 (2015) ix–x
http://dx.doi.org/10.1016/j.cvfa.2014.12.001
0749-0720/15/$ – see front matter © 2015 Published by Elsevier Inc.

high-quality, peer-reviewed guidance hardly meets our obligations as veterinarians. However, neither are our obligations met in a flurry of wizard-like potions based only on clinical impressions, physiologic extrapolation, or maybe just convention. Perhaps eliminating drugs from established protocols is a more challenging decision than adding new drugs.

The starting point in clinical decision-making is to understand the breadth and quality of available information. Toward that goal, the authors in this issue have completed rigorous, structured literature searches along with other means of locating information to bring a comprehensive review of available data to the clinician. Together, these authors are presenting concepts, data, and interpretations based on 465 references. Their searches took them through references numbering many times this amount, with methods for excluding papers that did not meet the standards of their articles. The next step for the clinician, as described in the article by Drs O'Connor and Fajt, is to become a discriminating consumer of this information.

On a personal note, we all have our personal journeys that have developed a passion within us to dig into an area of veterinary practice. For me, it was on a road between Macksville and Larned, Kansas, in 1989, returning from a call to help out on a disastrous respiratory disease outbreak in some high-risk calves. I made the decision about 15 miles south of Larned to leave practice with my father and enter a graduate program in clinical pharmacology to figure out a way to keep the calves from dying. Obviously, I have not been successful, and my article with Dr DeDonder is the culmination, but not the end, of 25 years of struggling to understand what antimicrobials actually do for us in bovine respiratory disease. Dr DeDonder is my current doctoral student and resident-in-training to sit for the American College of Veterinary Clinical Pharmacology (ACVCP) board examination; four other ACVCP Diplomates in this issue have preceded him (Drs Fajt, Wagner, Coetzee, and Lubbers). Seeing their contributions to this issue as well as to student and continuing education, professional service, research, and leadership in the profession is a privilege and a pleasure.

Michael D. Apley, DVM, PhD, DACVCP
Department of Clinical Sciences
Kansas State University College of Veterinary Medicine
111B Mosier Hall
Kansas State University
Manhattan, KS 66506, USA

E-mail address:
mapley@vet.ksu.edu

Evaluating Treatment Options for Common Bovine Diseases Using Published Data and Clinical Experience

CrossMark

Annette O'Connor, MVSc, DVSc, FANZCVSc[a], Virginia Fajt, DVM, PhD[b],*

KEYWORDS

- Comparative efficacy • Effect size • Study design • Clinical experience

KEY POINTS

- Not all sources of information provide unbiased estimates of treatment effects, and transparent sources that enable the assessment of biases are important when assessing treatments.
- Well-executed randomized controlled trials and systematic reviews of well-executed randomized controlled trials provide transparent unbiased comparison of treatment effects.
- Confounding by indication is a major source of bias in cohort studies and clinical experience.
- Case series and case reports provide no comparative assessment, and bias cannot be assessed, so provide little information for assessing the effect of treatments.
- Reports of comparative efficacy should provide an estimate of the magnitude of the effect size, including the precision of the effect size given by the 95% confidence interval; such information enables clinicians to better assess interventions than P values.

INTRODUCTION

This issue of *Veterinary Clinics of North America: Food Animal Practice* includes discussions and recommendations for the treatment of common bovine diseases, such as how to evaluate and diagnose each condition, select treatment options, and assess the outcome. Veterinarians have an obligation to provide treatment options based on the most recent research evidence tempered by clinical experience and the clinical setting (ie, the unique needs of the patients and client). In this article, the authors

The authors have nothing to disclose.
[a] Veterinary Medical Research Institute, College of Veterinary Medicine, Iowa State University, Building 4, Ames, IA 50010, USA; [b] Veterinary Physiology and Pharmacology, Texas A&M University College of Veterinary Medicine & Biomedical Sciences, 4466 TAMU, College Station, TX 77843-4466, USA
* Corresponding author.
E-mail address: vfajt@cvm.tamu.edu

Vet Clin Food Anim 31 (2015) 1–15
http://dx.doi.org/10.1016/j.cvfa.2014.11.001
0749-0720/15/$ – see front matter © 2015 Elsevier Inc. All rights reserved.

provide guidelines for evaluating sources of information, such as summaries of research, published primary research, and clinical experience. External sources of data should be used as sources of (1) estimates of treatment effect (in numerical form) and (2) precision of the treatment effect estimate, although the value of this information should be assessed in light of the risk of bias.

In addition to discussing how the magnitude and precision of the treatment effect are calculated, the authors discuss the risk of bias for all these sources. The authors use a framework that focuses on applicability and validity. Their basic approach is to introduce the external information sources available to veterinarians and how to evaluate them, and then to discuss how clinical experience should be evaluated. The discussion is limited to information that clinicians might use in the decision-making process about selecting treatment options. The approaches to assessing relevance and validity may not always directly apply to other clinical decisions, such as selecting preventive interventions or diagnostic tests for disease detection.

TREATMENT EFFICACY VERSUS CLINICAL DECISION MAKING

Here the authors draw the clear, but often ignored, distinction between deciding the effect of the treatment and deciding which treatment to use. To discuss this issue, the authors consider the situation when a clinician is faced with 3 treatment options: treatment A, treatment B, and the placebo group (no treatment). The clinician may find that treatment A reduced retreatments by 60%, whereas treatment B reduced retreatments by only 40%, when both are compared with a placebo. Clearly, treatment A is more effective. However, knowledge of the magnitude of effect does not mean the clinician will use treatment A. As frequently discussed, the setting must be considered. There is always an upper limit to the amount a producer can spend on treatments. If treatment A is 10 times more expensive than treatment B, in the face of an outbreak, the clinician might use the magnitude of the effect of treatment A and treatment B combined with the setting information (resources) to decide to treat 10 times as many animals with treatment B. Alternatively, if the same clinician is faced with treating just one animal that is a prized stud animal, the decision reached will likely be in favor of treatment A. These examples illustrate that the clinical setting combined with efficiency determine the treatment decisions, not solely the magnitude of the treatment effect.

WHAT INFORMATION IS NEEDED TO DETERMINE COMPARATIVE EFFICACY?

All decisions about treatments are comparative. If there is no comparison or alternatives to choose between, then there is no decision to make. When deciding on treatments, it is usual that a comparison is being made between treatment A and treatment B or even treatment C. Sometimes one of the treatments is to do nothing, which, in research, is often represented by the placebo group. Some studies will not include a placebo if it is considered unethical to leave animals untreated. Given this setting of a comparison, to make judgments about which treatment is most effective, 3 pieces of information are needed.

The Magnitude of the Effect Size

The magnitude of the effect size refers to how big the difference in the treatments is. Frequently, studies compare treatments on 2 effect size scales: the *mean difference* and the *risk ratio*.

The *mean difference* is used to describe the difference in means for continuous outcomes compared across treatments, such as weight gain or milk production. As this is a subtraction, mean differences can be negative or positive. If the treatments do not differ in effect, then the value of the mean difference would be zero (if there was no variation caused by sampling). **Table 1** shows some hypothetical examples of treatment comparisons. In the examples in the second, third, and fourth rows, the magnitude of the mean difference in treatments is the same, (ie, 4 units different). (For continuous outcomes, it is also possible to measure the effect size as the standardized mean different or ratio of means; but these are not discussed here.)

The *risk ratio* describes the ratio of risk for events. As with any ratio of 2 proportions, the risk ratio can vary from zero to infinity. If the two treatments do not affect the risk of disease, then the risk ratio would be one. Ratios bigger than one suggest the numerator has a high risk of the event; ratios less then one suggest the numerator has a lower risk than the denominator. It is not possible to write general rules about positive or negative effects based on a ratio greater than or less than one, because this depends if the event measured is considered a good or poor outcome. In the example in the fifth and sixth rows of **Table 1**, the magnitude of the risk ratio in treatments is the same (ie, 1.4), suggesting that the risk of the event is high in the treatment A group. If the event is recovery, this suggests treatment A has a higher recovery rate. If the event is adverse, such as retreatment, this suggests treatment A had a higher retreatment rate. Other outcomes that may be compared using ratios are prevalence and survival.

Notice from the 2 aforementioned examples that it is not possible to create effect size without a comparison, as is discussed later; this is why case reports and cases series are not useful for understanding treatment effects.

The Precision of the Effect Size

The precision refers to how precisely the magnitude of the effect size is known. Precision is often expressed as a 95% confidence interval, although other size intervals can be used. A narrow 95% confidence interval gives greater confidence in an effect size compared with a wider 95% confidence interval. The confidence interval is a function of the variation in the underlying study population and the sample size. For example, in the second and third rows of **Table 1**, the variation of the populations (shown by the standard deviation) is the same; however, the sample sizes in the studies differ, so the effect size from the study with the larger study size is known with greater precision. On the other hand, comparing the data in the third and fourth rows of **Table 1**, the magnitude of the effect size is the same and the sample size is the same, but the underlying variation in the population is affecting how precisely we know the estimate.

How to use confidence intervals in clinical decision making is difficult, but the goal is to consider the magnitude of the effect size and how well that effect size is known. For example, if a clinician was presented with study data similar to that in the second row of **Table 1**, he or she might conclude that treatment A is possibly more effective than treatment B (if the event is a positive event). However, if the same clinician was presented with the data in the third and fourth rows of **Table 1** he or she may have greater certainty about the superiority of treatment A and be less inclined to look for alternatives.

Finally, usually systematic reviews with meta-analyses provide more precise estimates of effect sizes, as these reviews are combining data across more studies. For example, in **Fig. 1**, there is a meta-analysis using the data from **Table 1**. The precision of the summary effect size is described by the 95% confidence interval, represented by the outer edges of the diamond in **Fig. 1**, and ranges from 1.63 to 6.49, which is narrower than any single study.

The P Value

Finally, most statistical analysis provides an estimate of the P value. The P value is a measure of the probability that you would see an effect as big or bigger than that observed in

Table 1
Hypothetical data from 5 studies comparing treatment A with treatment B: 2 types of outcome are presented, a continuous outcome (ADG) and risk of an event

Design	Treatment A Mean (SD)	Treatment B Mean (SD)	Effect Measure	Effect Size	95% CI of Effect Size	P Value
ADG (35 animals per group)	111.5 (9)	107.44 (9)	Mean difference	4.1	−0.23 to 8.35	.063
ADG (50 animals per group)	111.5 (9)	107.44 (9)	Mean difference	4.1	0.53 to 7.67	.025
ADG (50 animals per group)	111.5 (18)	107.44 (18)	Mean difference	4.1	−3.04 to 11.24	.257
Risk of event (50 animals per group)	10 of 50 (20)	7 of 50 (14)	Risk ratio	1.429	0.59 to 3.45	.44
Risk of event (500 animals per group)	100 of 500 (20)	70 of 500 (14)	Risk ratio	1.429	1.08 to 1.88	.01

Abbreviations: ADG, average daily gain; CI, confidence interval.

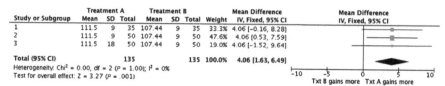

Study or Subgroup	Treatment A			Treatment B			Weight	Mean Difference IV, Fixed, 95% CI	Mean Difference IV, Fixed, 95% CI
	Mean	SD	Total	Mean	SD	Total			
1	111.5	9	35	107.44	9	35	33.3%	4.06 [-0.16, 8.28]	
2	111.5	9	50	107.44	9	50	47.6%	4.06 [0.53, 7.59]	
3	111.5	18	50	107.44	9	50	19.0%	4.06 [-1.52, 9.64]	
Total (95% CI)			135			135	100.0%	4.06 [1.63, 6.49]	

Heterogeneity: Chi² = 0.00, df = 2 (P = 1.00); I² = 0%
Test for overall effect: Z = 3.27 (P = .001)

Txt B gains more   Txt A gains more

Fig. 1. A forest plot using hypothetical data from 3 studies comparing treatment A with treatment of a continuous outcome (average daily gain). This example has no heterogeneity in effect size across studies. Chi², chi-square; CI, confidence interval; IV, inverse variance; Txt, treatment.

this study in a population whereby the mean difference was truly 0. Some people use the P value as a decision rule, (ie, if the P value is less than .05, the treatment is effective; if it is greater than .05, the treatment is ineffective). This approach is overly simplistic and strongly discouraged for interpreting study data. As can be seen in **Table 1**, the P value is also a confounded measure that is a function of magnitude of the effect, variation in the underlying population, and the sample size. Of course it is difficult to ignore a P value of .2.

If presented with only one study, the authors would argue that it is far better to look at the magnitude of effect and confidence interval and understand that these data suggest a possible effect but have uncertainty than to use the P value as a decision rule. The fact that some research summaries calculate a summary effect size from multiple studies, whether or not P values are mentioned, means that research summaries better describe the effect of the intervention.

WHAT ARE EXTERNAL SOURCES OF INFORMATION ABOUT TREATMENT OPTIONS?

Where should clinicians find information about comparative efficacy (ie, the magnitude of effect size, the precision of effect size and the P value)? Most, but not all, sources of external information are in the form of published studies, reports, or reviews. However, not all sources provide the magnitude of the effect sizes or the precision of the effect size of the P value; further, some sources might provide biased estimates of the effect size. External sources of information can be summaries of prior research (systematic reviews, narrative reviews, opinion) or primary research (trials, observational studies, case series, and case reports). External sources of information differ in their applicability to the clinician's decision and potential to produce valid (unbiased) estimates of the effect size. However, before validity and applicability is discussed, the authors briefly introduce sources of information.

Research Summaries Approaches

In the area of research summaries, common types of summaries are systematic reviews, narrative reviews, and opinion.

Systematic reviews with meta-analysis

A systematic review of randomized controlled trials (RCTs) is a summary of trials that compare one treatment to another treatment.[1-3] When a systematic review includes a meta-analysis, a magnitude of effect size is calculated, as is a precision estimate and a P value; explicit assessment of variation and sources of variation can be assessed. **Figs. 1** and **2** illustrate 2 meta-analyses; both calculate a summary measure of effect size, a measure of precision (the 95% confidence interval of the effect size), and an assessment of heterogeneity. In **Figs. 1** and **2**, the summary effect size is 4.1 and precision is the same 95% (1.6–6.5). However, the explicit assessment of heterogeneity based on the chi-square test for heterogeneity ($P = 1$ in **Fig. 1** and $P = .0001$ in **Fig. 2**) and I² (0% in

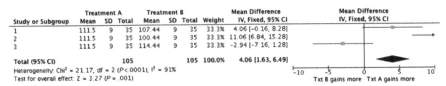

Fig. 2. A forest plot using hypothetical data from 3 studies comparing treatment A with treatment of a continuous outcome (average daily gain). This example has substantial heterogeneity in effect size across studies. Chi², chi-square; CI, confidence interval; IV, inverse variance.

Fig. 1 and 91% in **Fig. 2**) illustrates that the findings included in the review associated with **Fig. 1** are consistent, whereas the results from the second review are very variable (heterogeneous). Therefore, because the reporting is comprehensive, the end user has the option to either use the summary effect or ignore it based on the evidence of wide variation (heterogeneity of effect). Characteristics of well-executed systematic reviews include

- An a priori protocol defining the review process
- A specific question based on a population, interventions, and outcome
- A comprehensive search
- Explicit eligibly criteria
- Explicit extraction of outcome data
- Explicit assessment of presence of and sources of heterogeneity
- Explicit assessment of risk of bias within studies
- Explicit assessment of bias across studies
- Calculation of a summary effect size and precision of that estimate

It is possible to have a systematic review without a meta-analysis. Such reviews are useful because they include transparency about information sources and assessment of risk of bias; however, the absence of an effect size is a limitation.

Narrative reviews
Narrative reviews are often found in book chapters, journals, or continuing education (CE) proceedings.[3] These reviews often include data from numerous studies, but the rationale for inclusion of studies is often not justified. Usually the magnitude of the treatment effect is not calculated, and so the effect of the treatment is less clear. For example, a narrative review may report that treatment A was found to be superior to treatment B in one group but may not report or combine the magnitude of the effects. Also, in a narrative review, the presence of wide variation in outcomes and the source of that variation is often not explicitly discussed or assessed. It is often impossible to determine if the body of work being reviewed in a narrative review is consistent with the review in **Fig. 1** or **Fig. 2**, as narrative reviews rarely explicitly address heterogeneity.

It is of course possible that a narrative review is based on an extensive search of the literature and includes assessment of the risk of bias in the relevant studies; however, currently this is rare in veterinary science. Narrative reviews that include this information would be of more value that those that do not.

Opinion
Opinion is a common source of information about treatment options that can be oral (a phone or conference presentation) or written (on a blog or electronic list). Here the authors differentiate opinion from narrative reviews and reports written by experts, by the absence of references in opinions. Opinions usually do not report the magnitude of effect, the precision of the effect or a *P* value, or assess the presence of (or sources of)

variation (heterogeneity). Of course in an opinion, it is impossible to determine if the body of work being used to form the opinion is consistent like that in **Fig. 1** or has huge variation such as the situation in **Fig. 2**. Opinions expressed at conferences, in e-mail lists, or in phone consultations may be 100% accurate; however, this cannot be formally assessed. Therefore, another major issue with opinion is that it is not transparent. When an opinion is offered, it is not possible to differentiate between numerous possible scenarios, such as the opinion arises

- From inclusion of all relevant data, assessment of biases, and source of heterogeneity and, therefore, equals a systematic review
- From the selective assessment of a limited number of studies and is inadvertently biased
- From a conflict of interest whereby the expert may profit from the advice through increased sales, job security, consulting contracts, and so on and is biased

Primary Research Approaches

Randomized controlled trials

RCTs of treatments start with naturally occurring diseases in populations and are able to calculate a magnitude of effect, a precision estimate, and a P value.[4,5] The design has the following features:

- Random allocation to group: designed to enable the groups to be comparable; therefore, differences observed are attributed to the differs in treatment
- Blinding of allocation: prevents differences in treatment allocations
- Blinding of caregiving: prevents differential care that might bias the comparison
- Blinding of outcome assessment: prevents differential outcome assessment that might bias the comparison.

The use of naturally occurring disease populations is what differentiates an RCT from an experiment, which uses induced disease that may not be very applicable (see later discussion).

Cohort studies

Cohort studies are a common design in the published veterinary literature and are often misreported as a case series.[6–8] For treatment efficacy assessment, this design commonly arises from a retrospective evaluation of clinic/hospital records. The essential features are a group of animals with the disease of interest as the starting population and that this group received a variety of treatments based on clinical decisions; therefore, allocation to group is not random. The outcomes of those treatment groups are compared. Cohort studies can report effect size, the precision of the effect size, and the P value; however, these designs are subject to biases, in particular confounding by indication and loss to follow-up (see discussion below on validity).

Case series and case reports

These designs serve little purpose in assessing the efficacy of treatments, as no comparison groups exists, so no effect size can be estimated. A case series reports the outcome of a series of cases, and a case report reports the outcome of one case. Given the lack of comparison, each characteristic of the animals is confounded by treatment; therefore, no inference about treatment effect can be drawn.

Pharmacokinetics studies

Studies examining drug concentrations in cattle over time are relatively easy to perform, so many have been published. These studies do not provide any comparative information about treatments. Further, knowledge of drug concentrations in animals in the absence of a correlated response is impossible to interpret. Therefore, in order to be useful, pharmacokinetic studies cannot be viewed in a vacuum but must be interpreted in light of pharmacodynamic data. For example, drug concentration data for an antibiotic can be very useful if the minimum inhibitory concentrations of a population of bacterial isolates are known, although it must be considered that the interaction of the antibiotic and the pathogen may be quite different at the site of the infection. In the context of inferring treatment effect, however, pharmacokinetic studies alone are not useful; even when combined with in vitro pharmacodynamic data, the treatment effect is difficult to extrapolate. These studies may provide useful hypotheses for designing studies that can actually measure the treatment effect.

In vitro studies

As with pharmacokinetic studies, studies of in vitro effects of drugs cannot be interpreted as stand-alone data sets. If they are viewed in combination with pharmacokinetic data, however, they may be somewhat valuable in generating hypotheses about a potential treatment effect.

WHAT SHOULD I LOOK AT IN EXTERNAL INFORMATION SOURCES TO DETERMINE IF IT IS APPLICABLE AND VALID?

Table 2 summarizes the major sources of information as well as the ability of sources to provide the effect size, the precision of effect size, the risk of bias, and the ability to assess bias.[9]

WHAT IS MEANT BY APPLICABILITY AND WHAT FACTORS AFFECTED APPLICABILITY?

When an information source is applicable, it generally implies that we expect that the source would provide results that apply to the clinical decision-making setting. The

Table 2
Sources of information and the potential for risk of bias, ability to assess the risk of bias, and precision of the effect estimate

Evidence Type	Primary Research or Research Summary	Potential for Risk of Bias	Ability to Assess the Risk of Bias	Estimate of Treatment Effect Calculated	Precision of the Effect Estimate
Systematic review with meta-analysis of RCT	Summary	Low	High	Yes	High
Narrative review	Summary	High	Low	No	Not applicable
Opinion	Summary	High	Low	No	Not applicable
Large RCT	Primary	Low	High	Yes	High
Small RCT	Primary	Low	High	Yes	Low
Cohort study	Primary	High	Low	Yes	High
Case series	Primary	High	Low	No	Not applicable
Case reports	Primary	High	Low	No	Not applicable
Pharmacokinetic studies	Primary	Unclear	Unclear	No	Not applicable
In vitro studies	Primary	Unclear	Unclear	No	Not applicable

most important factors that affect the applicability of external information sources are the relevance of the population, outcome, and comparison.

Relevant Population

It is important to evaluate the description of the study population and determine if it is likely to be relevant to the target population. Clinicians should consider if the factors that differ between the study and target populations change the treatment effect. For example, a clinician is working with housed beef cattle in the Midwest United States and has 2 papers available that relate to the treatments being compared. One study was conducted in beef cattle in an Argentinian feedlot. The other study was conducted in housed dairy heifers in Canada. The studies available, therefore, differ from the target population in different ways: housing or production system. The clinician needs to decide which factor likely has the larger impact on the estimate of treatment effect. If he or she thinks that the production type has the greater effect, then the Argentinian paper should be used. If he or she decides that the housing system would have a greater impact on the treatment effect, then the study conducted in dairy cattle will be of greater relevance. In published reports, it is possible to assess the study population, which enables a judgment based on clinical expertise. With oral expert opinion, it is difficult to determine if the populations that form the basis for the opinion are applicable to your target population. This lack of transparency is one reason why this information source ranks poorly.

Relevant Outcomes

Some outcomes are more relevant than others. Factors that affect the value of an outcome are the relevance of the metric to the owner/clinician and repeatability of the metric. In livestock, the authors would propose that generally the following hierarchy of outcomes might apply to most situations:

- Production metrics: rate of gain, milk production, death
- Disease metrics: recovery, relapse rates, validated pain scores
- Proxy metrics: antibodies or bioavailability, biochemical markers for inflammation or pain or stress, culture results, susceptibility/resistance

This list is based on the concept that some outcomes are more relevant to the owner/clinician than others. If given the choice of a well-executed randomized trial that assessed body weight gain 5 weeks after treatment in calves diagnosed with bovine respiratory disease compared with a well-executed randomized trial that compared recovery of putative pathogens from the noses of calves 3 weeks after treatment, it is likely that, for assessing treatment, the weight gain is far more relevant to the owner and clinicians.

When evaluating the study result or result of research summary, the clinician should determine if the outcome is relevant or the combination of outcomes is valid in the case of a research synthesis. For example, if a clinician is interested in treatment success over 120 days and the data provided are only from a 10-day study, the study results may not be relevant. In research summaries, a well-reported meta-analysis should define the eligibility criteria of studies, including case definitions. The clinician is able to determine if he or she thinks the outcomes in the studies are relevant, comparable, and should be combined. Again, here is the advantage of the research synthesis methods that include transparent reporting of the eligibly criteria of studies included in the synthesis. The transparency of reporting the eligible studies enables assessment of relevance and bias. Narrative reviews and opinion deflect such scrutiny by providing no information about eligibility of studies or by not defining the explicit outcomes considered or assessment of heterogeneity.

Relevant Comparison Group

External information sources should have a comparison group; however, not all comparison groups are created equal. Clinicians likely have a comparison in mind when choosing a therapy, often a standard therapy compared with a new therapy. Clearly, a report that makes the comparison of interest is more relevant to the client or owner than a trial that compares a therapy against a negative control (unless a negative control is the current standard of practice). Although it is possible to make naïve indirect comparisons, these are often biased because of differences in baseline risk and study populations.

WHAT IS MEANT BY A VALID (UNBIASED) ESTIMATE OF THE EFFECT SIZE AND WHAT FACTORS AFFECTED VALIDITY (RISK OF BIAS)?

Threats to validity are numerous in external information sources. The aim is to obtain a valid estimate of the effect size. Some sources cannot provide a valid estimate because they do not include a comparison group. Other sources are able to provide an effect size, but biases may mean it is not valid. Next the common threats to validity that influence the ranking of external information sources are discussed.

The Inclusion of a Relevant Comparison Group

Although not technically a source of validity, information sources should have a comparison group, as this is essential to assessing treatment efficacy. Systematic reviews of RCTs, single RCTs, experiments that use challenge models, and cohort studies all include comparison groups. Case series and case reports do not. Depending on the narrative review, the mix of studies included may or may not be limited to those that include a comparison. For opinion, the role of case reports and cases series in the opinion cannot be determined.

Exchangeability of Comparison Groups

As discussed, a comparison group is a key feature for validity and systematic reviews of RCT, single RCT, experiments that use challenge models, and cohort studies. These designs, however, do not provide equally valid effect size estimates because for some designs the treatment groups are not exchangeable (ie, the treatment groups differ by characteristics other than the treatment that affects the outcome). Lack of randomization has been shown to be associated with biased estimates of treatment effects in numerous fields of study, including large animals.[10,11] A particular cause of nonexchangeability is confounding by indication.[7,8] The easiest example of confounding by indication is a cohort study based on hospital records. The reason animals receive a particular treatment is likely influenced by the clinician, and the clinician's decision in turn is influenced by prognostic factors.

Random allocation to a group is the key to comparability of groups provided a sufficient sample size is used (something like >30 animals).[12] Studies that can use randomization include systematic reviews, RCTs, and experiments; these, therefore, tend to have a lower risk of bias and, hence, greater internal validity when describing the effect of the treatments.

The main source of bias in cohort studies is confounding by indication, that is, animals with better expected outcomes are more likely to receive a particular treatment. Random allocation to group prevents this from occurring in RCTs. Because of confounding by indication, cohort studies have a higher risk of bias and rank lower than RCTs. Note that some might suggest that a large cohort study is of greater value than a small RCT. A small RCT would provide an unbiased estimate of the treatment effect with low precision, although a large cohort study likely provides a precise biased estimate of the treatment effect. It is preferable to have an imprecise correct estimate than a systematically biased estimate even if precisely estimated.

Repeatable Metrics of Outcomes

As the outcome is going to be compared across groups, it is important to look for an outcome that is not prone to subjective measurement. Death and weight gain are good examples of objective outcomes. If the outcome is prone to subjective measurement, then look for methods used to blind the outcome assessor to the treatment group. Failure to blind is associated with biased estimates of effect.[10,11,13] Blinding does not solve poor measurement but aims to make the extent of poor measurement equal across treatment groups. If the outcome is subjective and the person measuring the outcomes knows the treatment groups, the comparison across groups is subject to bias.

The reliability of measurement of a metric also influences its value in clinical decision making. For example, the alleviation of pain is a highly relevant outcome. However, some studies may use approaches to quantifying pain that are not validated. Similarly, the sensitivity and specificity of producer observation as a measure of *recovery*, or the opposite *failure*, may be subjective and not repeatable.

Given the choice between 2 equally powered RCTs, one of which compared recovery based on producer observation across 2 treatments and another that compared death across the two treatments, it is likely that measurement of death is more accurate than measurement of recovery, and so it might be given more weight in the clinical decision-making process.

Every Animal That Started the Study Finished the Study

It is important to know that all (or most) animals that started the study finished the study and data are available on them. If data are only used on a limited subset of animals for which outcomes are available, then the comparison reported might not reflect the comparison that occurred in the original group of animals.

Loss-to-follow-up bias is a threat to validity for case reports, case series, cohort studies, RCTs, and experiments. Studies with high loss to follow-up have been associated with biased estimates of treatment effect size.[14] In hospital record–based cohort studies and case reports/series, it is frequent that not all the outcomes are available on all treated patients. This information should be clear in the eligibility criteria. The investigators should report how many animals received the treatments and for how many treated animals the outcomes are available. This information allows for assessment of the potential for bias, although not the direction. Often, however, cohort studies and case series define the study population as animals with outcomes available. When this approach to defining the study population is used, loss to follow-up is no less of a threat to validity but it is less obvious because of the way the study eligibility was defined.

WHAT ABOUT CLINICAL EXPERIENCE: IS IT APPLICABLE AND VALID?

Recall that previously the authors discussed how vitally important knowledge of the clinical setting is to making valid clinical decisions about treatments. The authors illustrated the difference between deciding the effect of treatments (ie, the magnitude of the effect size) and deciding which treatment to use. In the next section, the authors discuss the limitations of clinical experience for measuring the effect size; again they emphasize that this is not the same as clinical decision making. Clinical experience is discussed using the same applicability and validity framework used for external information sources.

APPLICABILITY OF CLINICAL EXPERIENCE FOR DETERMINING THE EFFECT SIZE, THE PRECISION, AND THE *P* VALUE

Clearly, the great strength of clinical experience is the applicability of that experience to the current clinical decision. When drawing from clinical experience, the clinician's client base is far closer to the target population than any study, synthesis, or expert opinion can ever be. In some situations, the clinician's prior experience may come from working with the same farm environment or animals. That framework to understand how treatments have worked previously is invaluable. Even when working with an entirely new client, the veterinarian's client base has resulted in years of clinician experience that is likely more applicable to the new client than any study population in an external source.

VALIDITY OF CLINICAL EXPERIENCE FOR DETERMINING THE EFFECT SIZE, THE PRECISION AND THE *P* VALUE

Despite the very high applicability of clinical experience, there are possible issues with validity. However, the extent to which these validity issues are important varies across clinicians, clients, and clinics. Here the authors point out the potential threats to validity that can occur for clinical experience. Each clinician should examine these and determine how likely they are to bias their clinical experience and assessment of how effective a treatment is. Further discussions of sources of cognitive bias related to medical decision making are available.[15]

Lack of a Comparison Group

Lack of a comparison group is a potential source of bias in clinical experience. Some clinicians use the same therapy each time, which means that there is no comparison. In such circumstances, it is not possible to determine based on clinical experience if alternative treatments would perform better, worse, or equally well. This situation is even the case with 100% successful treatments. In such situations, it is possible without comparison that failure to apply any treatment would also result in 100% success.

Confounding by Indication Bias

As with any cohort study, the choice of which animal to allocate to a treatment is made by a clinician. More importantly, clinicians are by and large not making the decision randomly. Instead, the decision of which therapy to administer to an animal is based on prognostic factors and indicators to develop the best treatment. However, this of course means that the types of animals selected for different treatments differ and create confounding by indication. As with loss to follow-up (see later discussion), this is a major threat to validity. However, unlike loss to follow-up, there are few remedies to correct confounding by indication bias.

Loss to Follow-up

It is possible to think of clinical experience as one large cohort study built up over a career. Like any cohort study, clinical experience is likely very subject to loss-to-follow-up bias. As discussed, loss to follow-up is a major threat. Few clinicians are able to maintain records of outcomes from most treatments. Also, recall of case outcomes is likely imperfect. A professor of one of the author's once remarked that clinicians recall the 1st, the worst and the last case. There may be some truth in this statement, but regardless it is unlikely that clinicians either recall or have access to a census of outcomes or a random selection of outcomes. Therefore, although the cases seen are not biased and are highly applicable, the selection of cases for which outcomes are observed (or recalled) likely is.

As an extreme example, clinical experience can suffer dramatically from loss to follow-up. For example, perhaps a clinician uses 2 therapies. Over a 12-month period, the clinician treats 10 animals with treatment A and another 10 animals with treatment B. Further, to remove confounding by indication, let us imagine the clinician randomly allocated cases to the 2 treatments. In the follow-up period, the clinician is called to retreat 3 of the animals in the treatment B group and only 1 of the animals in the treatment A group. Based solely on these data, the clinician assumes treatment A is the superior treatment. However, the loss-to-follow-up data may tell a similar or very different story, as the number of scenarios that could have occurred in the other animals are almost boundless; this is why loss to follow-up is such a threat to validity of clinical experience. Next the authors give just 3 possible loss-to-follow-up scenarios.

- *Loss-to-follow-up scenario 1:* In the treatment A group, of the animals lost to follow-up, 1 animal recovered and the remaining 8 animals died. In the treatment group B, all the animals lost to follow-up recovered. In this case, B is truly the better therapy.
- *Loss-to-follow-up scenario 2:* In the treatment A group, all of the animals lost to follow-up recovered. In the treatment B group, 5 animals lost to follow-up recovered and 3 died. In this case, A is truly the better therapy.
- *Loss-to-follow-up scenario 3:* In the treatment A group, 6 of the animals lost to follow-up recovered, 1 animal was retreated by a different veterinarian, and 2 died. In the treatment B group, 6 of the animals lost to follow-up recovered and the remaining 2 died. In this case, the therapies are equal.

Loss to follow-up is a major reason why clinician impression/experience leads to potentially biased conclusions about efficacy. Few clinicians are able to follow up and discern the outcome from all patients. Also, the acquisition of information about cases is often not systematic. In some practices, it is possible that clients share positive outcomes more frequently and change vets when negative outcomes occur. Or perhaps, veterinarians learn more about negative outcomes because clients complain. The direction of the bias is unknown, making loss to follow-up so difficult to control. The extent to which loss to follow-up threatens the validity of clinical experience is based on the percentage of outcomes determined. In randomized trials, there is some discussion that losses of 20% to 30% may be acceptable; however, in cohort studies whereby allocation and loss to follow-up is rarely random, even low levels of loss to follow-up can create substantial biases.[16]

Biased Outcome Measurement

Another issue associated with clinical experience is the absence of blinding. Unfortunately, our perceptions of the outcome may be influenced by knowledge of the treatment. Of course, blinding is not possible with some outcomes, such as mortality; but outcomes such as recovery of function and client satisfaction can be biased by knowledge of the treatment. Further, if we seek the clients' opinions, their knowledge of the treatment received may also bias the assessment of the outcome.

SUMMARY

- Not all sources of information provide unbiased estimates of treatment effects.
- Transparent sources of research synthesis and primary research that enable the assessment of biases are important when assessing treatments.
- Well-executed RCTs and systematic reviews of well-executed RCTs provide transparent unbiased comparison of treatment effects.
- It is critical to evaluate each study or review to determine if it is well executed because publication is not a guarantee of quality. Ultimately, the responsibility for the assessment, applicability, and validity of each information sources lies with the end user.
- Confounding by indication is a major source of bias in cohort studies and clinical experience.
- Case series and case reports provide no comparative assessment, and bias cannot be assessed; so they provide little information for assessing the effect of treatments.
- Reports of comparative efficacy should provide an estimate of the magnitude of the effect size, including the precision of the effect size given by the 95% confidence interval. Such information enables clinicians to better assess interventions than *P* values.

REFERENCES

1. Higgins JP, Green S. Cochrane handbook for systematic reviews of interventions version 5.1.0. Oxford(UK): The Cochrane Collaboration; 2011.
2. Sargeant J, O'Connor AM. Introduction to systematic reviews in animal agriculture and veterinary medicine. Zoonoses Public Health 2014;61(Suppl 1):3–9.
3. O'Connor AM, Sargeant JM. An introduction to systematic reviews in animal health, animal welfare, and food safety. Anim Health Res Rev 2014;15:3–13.
4. O'Connor AM, Sargeant JM, Gardner IA, et al. The REFLECT statement: methods and processes of creating reporting guidelines for randomized controlled trials for livestock and food safety by modifying the CONSORT statement. Zoonoses Public Health 2010;57(2):95–104.
5. Sargeant JM, O'Connor AM, Gardner IA, et al. The REFLECT statement: reporting guidelines for randomized controlled trials in livestock and food safety: explanation and elaboration. Zoonoses Public Health 2010;57(2):105–36.
6. Sargeant JM, Kelton DF, O'Connor AM. Study designs and systematic reviews of interventions: building evidence across study designs. Zoonoses Public Health 2014;61(Suppl 1):10–7.
7. Valentine JC, Thompson SG. Issues relating to confounding and meta-analysis when including non-randomized studies in systematic reviews on the effects of interventions. Res Synth Methods 2013;4:26–35.
8. Wells GA, Shea B, Higgins JP, et al. Checklists of methodological issues for review authors to consider when including non-randomized studies in systematic reviews. Res Synth Methods 2013;4:63–77.
9. Sargeant JM, O'Connor AM. Conducting systematic reviews of intervention questions II: relevance screening, data extraction, assessing risk of bias, presenting the results and interpreting the findings. Zoonoses Public Health 2014; 61(Suppl 1):39–51.
10. Sargeant JM, Elgie R, Valcour J, et al. Methodological quality and completeness of reporting in clinical trials conducted in livestock species. Prev Vet Med 2009; 91:107–15.

11. Burns MJ, O'Connor AM. Assessment of methodological quality and sources of variation in the magnitude of vaccine efficacy: a systematic review of studies from 1960 to 2005 reporting immunization with Moraxella bovis vaccines in young cattle. Vaccine 2008;26:144–52.

12. Altman DG, Bland JM. How to randomise. BMJ 1999;319:703–4.

13. Sargeant JM, Thompson A, Valcour J, et al. Quality of reporting of clinical trials of dogs and cats and associations with treatment effects. J Vet Intern Med 2010;24: 44–50.

14. Guyatt GH, Oxman AD, Vist G, et al. GRADE guidelines: 4. Rating the quality of evidence–study limitations (risk of bias). J Clin Epidemiol 2011;64:407–15.

15. Croskerry P. From mindless to mindful practice–cognitive bias and clinical decision making. N Engl J Med 2013;368:2445–8.

16. Kristman V, Manno M, Cote P. Loss to follow-up in cohort studies: how much is too much? Eur J Epidemiol 2004;19:751–60.

Treatment of Mastitis in Cattle

Erin Royster, DVM, MS[a], Sarah Wagner, DVM, PhD[b],*

KEYWORDS

- Mastitis • Therapy • Antimicrobial • Evidence • Dairy • Cow • Lactating • Dry

KEY POINTS

- Treatment of mastitis is by common use of antimicrobial drugs in lactating and dry cows.
- Pathogen, cow, and drug factors should be considered when making mastitis treatment decisions.
- Evidence of clinical drug efficacy based on randomized, controlled clinical trials should be considered, if available, when choosing an antimicrobial drug for the treatment of mastitis.

INTRODUCTION

Drug treatment of mastitis during lactation remains common, as does treatment of cows at drying off. Our understanding of the disease, the causative pathogens, and the rationale for treatment or nontreatment under various circumstances continues to evolve. This article presents research-based evidence about the use or nonuse of drugs in cows with mastitis or at drying-off. Nondrug factors involved in decision making about mastitis, including cow characteristics and the epidemiology of mastitis, are also briefly discussed.

This article focuses on the use of antimicrobial drugs. Readers with an interest in the effects of anti-inflammatory drug treatment of cows with mastitis are referred to the excellent review by Leslie and Petersson-Wolfe, "Assessment and Management of Pain in Dairy Cows with Clinical Mastitis," published in 2012 in the *Veterinary Clinics of North America*.[1]

This article provides information that assists in the making of knowledgeable, evidence-based decisions about the therapy for mastitis. To that end, clinical trials of antimicrobial drugs for the treatment of mastitis in lactating and dry cows are presented and summarized. When reviewing this information, it is important to

The authors have nothing to disclose.
[a] Department of Veterinary Population Medicine, College of Veterinary Medicine, University of Minnesota, 225 Veterinary Medical Center, 1365 Gortner Avenue, Saint Paul, MN 55108, USA;
[b] Department of Animal Sciences, #7630, 1300 Albrecht Blvd., North Dakota State University, Fargo, ND 58108, USA
* Corresponding author.
E-mail address: Sarah.Wagner@ndsu.edu

Vet Clin Food Anim 31 (2015) 17–46
http://dx.doi.org/10.1016/j.cvfa.2014.11.010
vetfood.theclinics.com

remember that if a study is designed to detect treatment differences and fails to do so, this does not mean that the treatments are necessarily equally effective. For further discussion of this concept, see the article by Brian Lubbers elsewhere in this issue.

DETECTION AND DEFINITIONS

Mastitis is most frequently recognized in its clinical form, defined by the presence of visibly abnormal milk. Milk from a quarter with clinical mastitis may be watery or thickened and discolored with blood, pus, flakes, or clots (aka gargot). Cows with clinical mastitis may also experience swelling and redness or pain in the affected quarter and in some cases may become systemically ill with symptoms such as fever, dehydration, weakness, and inappetence. Clinical cases are designated as mild, moderate, or severe, corresponding to the presence or absence of local and systemic signs (**Table 1**). Recording the severity score of each case is helpful in evaluating prevention and detection practices, as well as treatment outcomes.

Although treatment of mastitis is mostly directed toward clinical cases, many cases of mastitis are subclinical, with no visibly detectable changes in milk. Subclinical mastitis infections are therefore identified by an elevated milk somatic cell count (SCC) in the affected quarter. An SCC in composite milk samples (milk from all 4 quarters) of greater than 200,000 cells/mL is commonly used to indicate that one or more quarters are infected. Cows with subclinical mastitis are often identified when the herd is tested through the Dairy Herd Improvement Association (DHIA), where milk SCC is measured in the laboratory, or by using an on-farm test to estimate the SCC. The most common cow-side test for subclinical mastitis is the California Mastitis Test (CMT). Identification and treatment of cows with subclinical mastitis may be a useful strategy to help reduce SCC in the farm bulk milk tank but is of equivocal economic benefit because of the costs of treatment and milk withdrawal and low treatment efficacy.[2–4] However, in herds in which contagious mastitis is an issue, identification and treatment of subclinically infected cows that are likely to respond to therapy may be advisable to decrease the risk of transmission.

It is important to evaluate the outcomes of any treatment or management action for mastitis to gauge success or failure. There are several outcomes following a case of mastitis that may be of interest to the practitioner or producer, including clinical or microbiological cure, days of milk withheld from sale, SCC, milk production, recurrence of mastitis, and retention in the herd.[5] Clinical cure is defined as a return to normal-appearing milk. The definition of microbiological cure varies considerably in the research literature depending on the method used to diagnose the causative pathogen (microbiological culture or other molecular diagnostic methods) and the sampling interval. Microbiological cure occurs when the organism originally identified as causing the infection cannot be isolated from the gland at some time point or points after treatment. Both these definitions of cure have strengths and weaknesses. Clinical cure is possible to evaluate on the farm and is one determinant of when milk can be returned to the saleable tank (the other being antibiotic drug withholding

Table 1	
Severity scoring system for mastitis	
Score	**Description**
1. Mild	Abnormal milk (eg, clots, flakes, watery)
2. Moderate	Abnormal milk and signs of udder inflammation (eg, heat, swelling, pain)
3. Severe	Systemic illness (eg, fever, dehydration, weakness, inappetence)

time) but may be confounded by the fact that some infections revert to a subclinical state after or regardless of treatment. Microbiological cure cannot usually be evaluated on-farm and is therefore impractical for most mastitis cases but may be a more accurate indicator of resolution of infection and a better predictor of other outcomes, such as reduction in SCC.[6] One or both of these definitions may be used in clinical trials designed to evaluate the efficacy of mastitis therapies. Clinical cure and outcomes such as milk production and SCC may be of greater interest to the producer, as these factors have a direct impact on the economics of the dairy and on management decisions.

ETIOLOGY

Mastitis, whether clinical or subclinical, is almost always caused by intramammary (IMM) infection (IMI) with bacteria. The bacteria that commonly cause mastitis are classified into contagious pathogens, which are transmitted from cow to cow on fomites at milking time, and environmental pathogens, which have their reservoir in the cows' environment.

Mycoplasma is a contagious pathogen that is not an uncommon cause of mastitis; a review article describes the frequency of isolation of *Mycoplasma* species in farm bulk milk tanks as varying from just more than 2% to more than 20% of herds, depending on herd size and geographic location, with larger, western herds having higher *Mycoplasma* prevalence.[7] However, mastitis caused by *Mycoplasma* is not responsive to drug treatment. Control strategies are directed at testing, segregation, and culling.

The other contagious pathogens, *Staphylococcus aureus* and *Streptococcus agalactiae*, have historically been among the most common causes of mastitis in dairy cows. A survey of milk cultures submitted to a diagnostic laboratory in the early 1980s found that the most common bacterial isolates were *S aureus* and *S agalactiae*, which together comprised 87% of isolates.[8] Similarly, composite (4-quarter) samples from more than 23,000 cows housed on 50 dairies in California in the 1980s yielded the same 2 pathogens most frequently.[9] Owing to the high prevalence of IMI due to *S aureus* and *S agalactiae* infection years ago, these 2 pathogens were historically the most frequent targets of drug therapy on dairy farms and of studies performed in pursuit of US Food and Drug Administration (FDA) approval of antimicrobial drugs for IMM therapy for mastitis.

The relative prevalence with which pathogens are isolated from cases of IMI has changed during the past 30 years. Within the last 10 years, cultured samples of 449 quarters from 422 cows in Minnesota, Wisconsin, and Ontario, housed on dairies ranging in size from 144 to 1795 cows, most commonly yielded coliform bacteria (24% of cases), non-*agalactiae* streptococci (14%), and coagulase-negative staphylococci (9%).[10] In that study, only 7% of isolates were *S aureus*, and none were *S agalactiae*. Similar results were obtained during a clinical trial in New York conducted in 2010 and 2011, which enrolled 296 cases of mastitis from 7 farms milking 357 to 1578 cows.[11] In that study, the most commonly isolated pathogen was *Streptococcus dysgalactiae,* followed by *Escherichia coli,* other esculin-positive cocci, *Streptococcus uberis,* and *Klebsiella* species.

The evidence suggests that efforts directed at controlling contagious mastitis have been largely successful and that as these efforts have succeeded, the predominant pathogens have become environmental, including coliforms and Gram-positive pathogens other than *S aureus* and *S agalactiae*. This situation complicates decision making about mastitis therapy, especially in the absence of microbial cultures of mastitis cases. Gram-negative pathogens have become far more common in the etiology of IMI, and some culture-based treatment programs recommend leaving cows with Gram-negative isolates on milk culture untreated.[10] However, a recent investigation[12] found that untreated cows with IMI due to Gram-negative pathogens had lower rates of clinical and microbiological cure and left the herd at a higher rate when compared with cows with IMI of Gram-negative causes treated with IMM antimicrobial therapy.

When culture information about a particular case of mastitis or the prevalent pathogens on the farm is unavailable, the most recent evidence about the prevalence of mastitis pathogens in the United States suggests that it is prudent to assume that the causative agent may be Gram-positive, Gram-negative, or *Mycoplasma* and to plan control, diagnosis, and treatment regimens accordingly.

CASE SELECTION—TO TREAT OR NOT TO TREAT?

With mastitis being the top reason for antibiotic use on dairies[13] and increasing scrutiny of the use of antibiotics in food animals, it is imperative that producers and practitioners follow best practices to use antibiotics selectively and judiciously. Several studies have identified characteristics or risk factors related to clinical mastitis and described their potential as predictors of outcomes or treatment success.[6,14–16] These factors include cow factors such as age or parity, stage of lactation (days in milk [DIM]), SCC, and clinical mastitis history, and pathogen factors such as virulence and antibiotic susceptibility. With these factors in mind, the first decision in a mastitis treatment protocol should be whether or not a particular case is eligible for antimicrobial drug therapy. Antimicrobial drug treatment should be reserved for cases that are likely to benefit from it, and cases that are extremely unlikely to benefit from treatment should be managed in other ways.

Much research on cow-level factors and the probability of cure for clinical mastitis cases has been focused on *S aureus*.[16–18] The findings of these studies were summarized by Barkema and colleagues.[19] Increasing parity, elevated SCC before treatment, and having multiple quarters affected were associated with a decreased probability of cure. In a study by Pinzón-Sánchez and Ruegg[5] of outcomes in mild or moderate clinical mastitis cases undifferentiated by causative pathogen, there was a tendency for decreasing probability of microbiological cure with increasing parity and a significant association between previous occurrence of clinical mastitis and decreasing microbiological cure. In this study, cases that experienced microbiological cure had a lower somatic cell score (the natural logarithm of SCC) at the DHIA test previous to the onset of mastitis compared with those that were not cured (3.1 vs 4.9, $P = .004$). These findings suggest that cow-level factors, including parity, history of infection, and previous SCC status, should be considered for all cases of clinical mastitis. Producers should also consider other cow-level factors that would affect the likelihood of a cow remaining in the herd long term before deciding to treat a case of mastitis. Cows that are later in lactation and not pregnant, sick with other concurrent illness, and lame or not producing much milk should be considered as potential cull candidates, rather than treatment candidates.

Differences in cure rates and other outcomes among mastitis pathogens have been well demonstrated.[5,14,20] For example, mastitis caused by pathogens such as *S aureus* and *S uberis* has lower cure rates compared with that caused by other species of staphylococci and streptococci. These differences may be explained by virulence factors specific to the organism, such as toxins produced, degree of tissue invasion or damage, and immunosuppression, or they may be due to differences in antimicrobial susceptibility. Within *S aureus* species, isolates that are positive for β-lactamase (a hydrolytic enzyme that deactivates β-lactam antibiotic drugs) are known to have much lower cure rates compared with isolates that are β-lactamase negative, even when the treatment used is not a β-lactam drug.[19] In the group of mastitis pathogens commonly referred to as environmental streptococci, there are differences in antibiotic susceptibility; for example, *Enterococcus* spp demonstrate more frequent resistance compared with other species in this group.[21] Although antibiotic susceptibility undoubtedly plays a role in response to therapy, there is little evidence of a correlation between in vitro susceptibility testing and treatment outcomes in the cow.[22] These differences in expected outcomes among mastitis pathogens should be considered when making treatment or management decisions for cases of clinical mastitis with the goal of reserving antimicrobial drug use for infections that are likely to benefit.

Combining knowledge of the pathogen causing infection with a cow's mastitis and SCC history is most informative for the decision maker in selecting an appropriate treatment or management action for a cow with clinical mastitis. This requires good record-keeping practices, whereby individual cow records include mastitis case history with date, severity score, and quarter affected, as well as test-day SCC. Knowledge of the pathogen causing infection has not typically been available for cow-side decision making, as results from mastitis culture performed off the farm at a diagnostic laboratory may take several days. However, the use of on-farm culture programs that use selective bacterial growth media to categorize cases of mastitis into broad diagnostic groups (such as no growth, Gram positive, or Gram negative) is increasing. With on-farm culture systems, results are typically available within 18 to 24 hours at a low cost. In mastitis cases in which no bacteria are isolated from milk culture, the use of IMM antimicrobials is not justified. No bacterial growth is found in 10% to 40% of clinical mastitis cases,[23,24] and when these cases are identified using on-farm culture, antimicrobial use may be greatly reduced.[10] Further, some producers may choose not to use an IMM antimicrobial drug for mild or moderate cases of mastitis caused by Gram-negative pathogens, as these infections have been shown to have a high rate of spontaneous cure.[2,25,26] Alternatively, some may choose to use a different IMM antimicrobial drug for mastitis of Gram-negative or Gram-positive origin to target the pathogen with a product that has an appropriate spectrum of activity.

In summary, mastitis treatment protocols should include eligibility criteria, and mastitis decision-makers should be trained to apply these selective criteria in every case. Cows that are unlikely to benefit from antimicrobial drug therapy because of infection with a difficult-to-cure pathogen or chronic infection should be managed in other ways or culled. Management options for cows that are not treated include segregation, drying off the infected quarter, or drying off the cow early. Drying off the quarter (either by cessation of milking or by chemically damaging the gland) is not without risks and should be reserved for cases in which the cow is otherwise healthy and productive.

INTRAMAMMARY TREATMENT WITH ANTIMICROBIAL DRUGS: LACTATING COWS

Cases of mastitis that occur during lactation are commonly treated using antimicrobial drugs manufactured and approved for IMM administration. Treatment of mastitis using antimicrobial drugs administered by other routes is not described here because there is no approval for any drug for such use by the FDA and such use is not typically a component of therapy for mild or moderate cases of mastitis. The focus in this article is on information published within the past 20 years, although older work is presented when nothing more current could be found. There is good reason to think that the most common pathogens now and the predominant pathogens 20+ years ago are not the same; this must be taken into account when weighing the utility of information from older clinical trials.

A retrospective study by Wilson and colleagues[3] offers some insight into the spontaneous cure rates for IMIs and the cure rates that may be achieved using IMM antimicrobial drug therapy. Because of the retrospective nature of the study, clinical severity could not be evaluated, so only subclinical cases were included in the analyses; this may have affected the observed outcomes. A case of mastitis was defined as microbial growth on a routine herd milk culture, and a cure was defined as no microbial growth on microbial culture the following month. Dosing regimens were not described. Twenty-one different pathogens were isolated from 9007 milk samples. The rate of spontaneous cure (without drug treatment) was 65% (4206/6481), whereas the rate of cure among cows treated with any antimicrobial drugs was 75% (1891/2526). The rate of elimination of IMI varied considerably by pathogen and drug. Based on the overall treatment data from this study, 10 cows would have to be treated with IMM antimicrobial drugs to effect one more cure than would be seen if no cows were treated. This number is calculated by dividing 100% by the percent reduction in bad outcomes (in this case, failure of the mastitis to resolve), and it is known as number needed to treat or NNT. In this case, because the number of uncured cases of mastitis is reduced by 10% with treatment, one would have to treat 10 cows to produce one more cure than one would observe without treatment.

Studies presented in this article as evidence to evaluate the efficacy of antimicrobial drug therapy in lactating cows are mostly limited to studies of naturally occurring mastitis in only 1 quarter and treating only that quarter, as cows with multiple affected quarters are less likely to experience a cure in any quarter.[19] In addition, the focus is on clinical expression of IMI; studies of subclinical disease are excluded when other good evidence is available. These limits are used to enhance the applicability of the evidence to decisions about the treatment of clinical mastitis and to maximize the similarity of research results presented for each antimicrobial agent.

Table 2 describes the antimicrobial preparations approved by the FDA for IMM administration to cows.

Tables 3 and **4** summarize clinical and microbiological outcomes of clinical trials of antimicrobial drugs approved for IMM administration to cows in the United States.

Beta-Lactams: Penicillins

Amoxicillin

Amoxicillin (Amoxi-Mast; New Animal Drug Application [NADA] 055-100) is an aminopenicillin with an expected spectrum of activity that includes Gram-positive bacteria that do not produce β-lactamase and some Gram-negative bacteria such as the Enterobacteriaceae, a family of bacteria that includes *E coli* and *Klebsiella* spp.

The package insert states that "Amoxi-Mast is indicated in the treatment of subclinical infectious bovine mastitis in lactating cows due to *Streptococcus agalactiae* and penicillin-sensitive *Staphylococcus aureus*." The label also claims "in vitro activity against alpha- and beta-hemolytic streptococci, nonpenicillinase-producing staphylococci, and *Escherichia coli*," whereas "most strains of *Pseudomonas*, *Klebsiella*, and *Enterobacter* are resistant." The label dose is 1 tube containing 62.5 mg amoxicillin IMM every 12 hours for 3 total treatments.[27]

Table 2
Antimicrobial products approved in the United States for intramammary treatment of lactating cows with mastitis

Name (Active Compound)	Label Indication	Dosage	Milk/Meat Withdrawal
Amoxi-Mast (62.5 mg amoxicillin)	S agalactiae, non–penicillin resistant S aureus (subclinical)	q 12 h for 3 consecutive treatments	60 h or 5 milkings/ 12 d meat
Dariclox (200 mg sodium cloxacillin)	S agalactiae, non–penicillin resistant S aureus	q 12 h for 3 consecutive treatments	48 h or 4 milkings/ 10 d meat
Hetacin-K (hetacillin potassium, 62.5 mg ampicillin activity)	S agalactiae, S dysgalactiae, S aureus, E coli	q 24 h for 3 consecutive treatments	72 h or 6 milkings/ 10 d meat
ToDay (200 mg cephapirin sodium)	S agalactiae, S aureus (including penicillin-resistant strains)	q 12 h for 2 consecutive treatments	96 h milk/4 d meat
Pirsue (50 mg pirlimycin hydrochloride)	Staphylococcus and Streptococcus spp	q 24 h, 2 to 8 consecutive days	36 h milk/9 d meat if 2 d of treatment; 21 d meat if treated >2 d
Spectramast (125 mg ceftiofur hydrochloride)	Coagulase-negative staphylococci, S dysgalactiae, E coli	q 24 h, 2 to 8 consecutive days	72 h milk/2 d meat

Check treatment information and milk and meat withdrawal times with drug manufacturer before prescribing based on this information.

Research done as part of the FDA approval process for Amoxi-Mast included one study with an untreated control group, evaluating treatment of mastitis due to S aureus and S agalactiae. Data from the approval study about S agalactiae are not presented here, as the pathogen is uncommon now and nearly universally susceptible to all IMM antimicrobial drug preparations on the market. Outcomes for cows with S aureus infection treated at the label dosage were as follows:

- "Freedom of Information Summary, Original New Animal Drug Application 055-100"[28]
  - Case definition: duplicate milk cultures isolating S aureus
  - Treatment groups
    - Untreated controls
    - Amoxicillin 62.5 mg IMM every 12 hours × 3
  - Cure definition: absence of the initial pathogen on duplicate cultures of the milk "approximately 23 days after treatment"
  - Treatment outcome differences: yes, treated group had more cure than untreated controls
  - Clinical cure rate: not reported
  - Microbiological cure rate
    - Untreated controls: 34% (18/53)
    - Amoxicillin: 81% (43/53)
  - NNT for 1 additional cure: 3 (2.12)
  - Comment: What the effect of treatment would be over a longer term is not known; this is an important consideration with S aureus as it is not uncommon for pathogen shedding to be reduced after treatment, then resume later.

Table 3
Clinical outcomes in trials of intramammary antimicrobial drug treatment of mastitis in lactating cows

Reference	Randomized?	Case Definition	Success Definition	N	Treatments	Positive Case Outcome (%)	Number Needed to Treat
Guterbock et al,[25] 1993	Yes	Abnormal milk appearance	Negative milk culture on day 8 and day 20	74 75 105	Amoxicillin 200 mg IMM q 12 h × 3 Cephapirin 200 mg IMM q 12 h × 2 Oxytocin 100 U IM q 12 h × 2–3	67.6 66.7 66.7	— — —
Roberson et al,[29] 2004	Yes	Abnormal milk ± 1 additional clinical sign	3 Consecutive normal milk observations or no relapse within 3 wk (evaluated days 1–8, 15, 22, 29, 36)	22 21 20 15	Untreated control Amoxicillin 200 mg IMM q 12 h × 3 Milking out q 2 h with oxytocin 20 U IM each time Combined amoxicillin and milking out as earlier	64.0 57.0 25.0 53.0	— — — —
Schukken et al,[11] 2013	Yes	Abnormal milk ± inflammation of udder	No clinical signs 10 d and 17 d after treatment	96 97	Cephapirin 200 mg IMM q 12 h × 2 doses Ceftiofur 125 mg IMM q 24 h × 5 d	Gram+: 65 Gram–: 50 Gram+: 62 Gram–: 44	— —
Ceftiofur FOI	Yes	Abnormal milk or udder inflammation and positive CMT result	Absence of pretreatment pathogen on milk culture 14 and 21 d after treatment	117 112	Untreated control Ceftiofur 125 mg IMM q 24 h × 2 d	54.7 78.6	— 3.44
Pirlimycin FOI: clinical and microbiological outcomes evaluated together	Yes	Abnormal milk ± inflammation of udder	Negative milk culture and normal milk 11 d after treatment	118 123	Untreated control Pirlimycin 50 mg IMM q 24 h × 2 d	28.0 48	— 5

Data from Refs.[11,25,30,36,39]

Table 4
Microbial outcomes in trials of intramammary antimicrobial drug treatment of mastitis in lactating cows

Reference	Randomized?	Case Definition	Success Definition	N	Treatments	Positive Case Outcome (%)	Number Needed to Treat
Guterbock et al,[25] 1993	Yes	Abnormal milk appearance	Negative milk culture on day 8 and day 20	74	Amoxicillin 200 mg IMM q 12 h × 3	43.9	—
				75	Cephapirin 200 mg IMM q 12 h × 2	55.0	—
				105	Oxytocin 100 U IM q 12 h × 2–3	49.1	—
Roberson et al,[29] 2004	Yes	Abnormal milk ± 1 additional clinical sign	3 Consecutive negative cultures or no relapse within 3 wk. (cultured days 1–8, 15, 22, 29, 36)	22	Untreated control	55.0	—
				21	Amoxicillin 200 mg IMM q 12 h × 3	67.0	—
				20	Milking out q 2 h with oxytocin 20 U IM each time milking out as earlier	45.0	—
				15	Combined amoxicillin and milking out as earlier	53.0	—
Rosenberg et al,[34] 2002	Yes	Positive CMT result on day 2 or 3 of lactation (subclinical)	No growth on microbial milk culture 2 and 4 wk after treatment	27	Untreated control	30.0	—
				19	Cephapirin 200 mg IMM q 12 h × 2	53.0	—
Schukken et al,[11] 2013	Yes	Abnormal milk ± inflammation of udder	Absence of pretreatment pathogen on milk culture 10 and 17 d after start of treatment	96	Cephapirin 200 mg IMM q 12 h × 2 doses	Gram+: 68 Gram−: 50	—
				97	Ceftiofur 125 mg IMM q 24 h × 5 d	Gram+: 67 Gram−: 79	—
Ceftiofur FOI	Yes	Abnormal milk or udder inflammation and positive CMT	Absence of pretreatment pathogen on milk culture 14 and 21 d after treatment	117	Untreated controls	41.3	—
				112	Ceftiofur 125 mg IMM q 24 h × 2 d	70.4	4.18
Oliver et al,[37] 2004	Yes	Subclinical SCC>400,000 2 milk cultures at 1-wk interval with same pathogens	Negative milk culture 14 and 28 d after treatment	38	Untreated controls	11	—
				49	Ceftiofur 125 mg IMM q 24 h × 2 d	39	3.6 (vs control)
				41	Ceftiofur 125 mg IMM q 24 h × 5 d	54	—
				38	Ceftiofur 125 mg IMM q 24 h × 8 d	66	4.5 (vs 2 doses)

Data from Refs.[11,25,30,35,36,38]

No results of prospective clinical trials treating naturally occurring clinical mastitis during lactation with amoxicillin could be found with publication dates in the last 20 years. Two older studies are summarized:

- "Efficacy of Intramammary Antibiotic Therapy for Treatment of Clinical Mastitis Caused by Environmental Pathogens" by Guterbock and colleagues[25]
  - Case definition: abnormal milk only
  - Treatment groups
    - Amoxicillin 200 mg IMM every 12 hours × 3
    - Cephapirin 200 mg IMM every 12 hours × 2
    - Oxytocin 100 U IM every 12 hours × 2 to 3
  - Cure definition
    - Clinical: normal milk appearance 8 days and 20 days after treatment
    - Microbiological: negative milk culture 8 days and 20 days after treatment
  - Treatment outcome differences: none statistically significant
  - Clinical cure rate
    - Amoxicillin 67.6% (50/74)
    - Cephapirin 66.7% (50/75)
    - Oxytocin 66.7% (70/105)
  - Microbiological cure rate
    - Amoxicillin: 43.9% (18/41)
    - Cephapirin: 55.0% (22/40)
    - Oxytocin: 49.1% (28/57)
  - NNT for 1 additional cure: N/A no untreated controls and no significant outcome differences
  - Comment: This study is unusual because of the similarity in outcomes for cases treated with antimicrobial drugs and cases treated without the use of antimicrobial drugs.
- "Mild to Moderate Clinical Mastitis: Efficacy of Intramammary Amoxicillin, Frequent Milk-out, a Combined Intramammary Amoxicillin, and Frequent Milk-out Treatment Versus no Treatment" by Roberson and colleagues[29]
  - Case definition: abnormal milk
    - Maximum 1 additional clinical sign (elevated temperature, heart rate or respiratory rate, decreased rumen contraction force, dehydration, or depression)
  - Treatment groups
    - Untreated control
    - Amoxicillin 200 mg IMM every 12 hours × 3
    - Milking out every 2 hours with oxytocin 20 U IM each time
    - Combined amoxicillin and milking out as earlier
  - Cure definition
    - Cows evaluated on days 1 to 8 after treatment began, also on days 15, 22, 29, and 36
    - Clinical: 3 consecutive evaluations with normal milk appearance or 2 weeks without relapse
    - Microbial: No growth on culture at 3 consecutive evaluations or 2 weeks without relapse
  - Treatment outcome differences: none statistically significant
  - Clinical cure rate
    - Untreated: 64% (14/22)
    - Amoxicillin: 57% (12/21)

- Milking out: 25% (5/20)
- Combined amoxicillin and milking out: 53% (10/19)
  ○ Microbiological cure rate
    - Untreated: 55% (12/22)
    - Amoxicillin: 67% (14/21)
    - Milking out: 45% (9/20)
    - Combined amoxicillin and milking out: 53% (10/19)
  ○ NNT for 1 additional cure: N/A no significant differences found
  ○ Comments: low statistical power to detect treatment differences

In summary, no recent studies evaluating the efficacy of amoxicillin for treating clinical mastitis could be found, and older studies had limited statistical power. Amoxicillin may or may not increase the rate of clinical or microbiological cure of mastitis in lactating cows under the conditions encountered at present.

Ampicillin (hetacillin)

Hetacillin (Hetacin-K; NADA 055-054) is rapidly transformed into ampicillin after administration and is therefore expected to have a spectrum of activity that is essentially the same as amoxicillin.

On the package insert, the drug indications are described as follows: "Hetacin-K for intramammary infusion has been shown to be efficacious in the treatment of mastitis in lactating cows caused by susceptible strains of *Streptococcus agalactiae*, *Streptococcus dysgalactiae*, *Staphylococcus aureus* and *Escherichia coli*." The label dose is 1 tube containing the equivalent of 62.5 mg ampicillin activity every 24 hours for a total of 3 treatments.[30]

Published results of clinical trials evaluating the efficacy of hetacillin for the treatment of clinical mastitis during lactation could not be found. It is similar to amoxicillin and is likely to have similar efficacy.

Cloxacillin

Cloxacillin (Dariclox; NADA 055-070) is a penicillinase-resistant penicillin that is expected to have a spectrum of activity that includes strains of *Staphylococcus* that produce β-lactamase. It has diminished efficacy against Gram-negative bacteria when compared with the aminopenicillins.

The package insert states that "Dariclox is indicated in the treatment of bovine mastitis in lactating cows due to *Streptococcus agalactiae* and nonpenicillinase-producing *Staphylococcus aureus*." The label dose is 1 tube containing 200 mg cloxacillin IMM every 12 hours for 3 doses.[31]

As with some of the other penicillins that have been available in the United States for a long time, recent (last 20 years) reports of clinical trials of naturally occurring cases of mastitis in lactating cows treated with cloxacillin could not be found. The most recent publications investigating treatment with IMM cloxacillin describe its use in pregnant heifers before the onset of their first lactation; the popularity of such applications seems mostly to have passed.

Shepard and colleagues[32] investigated the efficacy of cloxacillin in combination with systemic administration of erythromycin in recently calved cows with SCCs greater than 500,000 cells/mL of milk and found that clinical cure rates were lower for treated cows that for untreated controls. The investigators suspected that poor hygiene when introducing the drug into the mammary gland was responsible for this unexpected result.

In summary, there is a dearth of timely evidence to support or discourage the treatment of mastitis in lactating cows with cloxacillin.

Beta-Lactams: Cephalosporins

Cephapirin

Cephapirin (ToDay; NADA 097-222) is a member of the first-generation cephalosporin drug class and as such is expected to have a spectrum of activity that includes the Enterobacteriaceae and most Gram-positive bacteria, including β-lactamase-producing staphylococci.

Per the product label, ToDay "has been shown to be efficacious in the treatment of mastitis in lactating cows caused by susceptible strains of *Streptococcus agalactiae* and *Staphylococcus aureus* including strains resistant to penicillin." The label dosage is 1 tube containing 200 mg cephapirin activity IMM every 12 hours for 2 total doses.[33]

As with the penicillins, it has been decades since IMM cephapirin was first approved by the FDA for marketing in the United States. As with cloxacillin, many of the most recently published studies evaluating the effects of cephapirin examined its use in pregnant heifers and will not be described here.

In 2002, Rosenberg and colleagues[34] conducted a trial of cephapirin as a treatment for subclinical IMI in cows early in lactation. As the results of few clinical trials involving cephapirin have been published in the last 20 years, the results are summarized below.

- "Bacterial Cure and Somatic Cell Count Response of Dairy Cows with a Positive California Mastitis Test at Calving to Therapy with Cephapirin Sodium" by Rosenberg and colleagues[34]
  - Case definition: positive CMT on second or third day in milk
    - No depression, no rectal temperature greater than 40.6°C, no respiratory disease signs
    - No history of contagious mastitis
    - Not less than 3 functional teats
  - Treatment groups
    - Untreated control
    - Cephapirin 200 mg IMM every 12 hours × 2
  - Cure definition
    - No microbial growth on milk culture 2 and 4 weeks after treatment
  - Treatment outcome differences: higher microbiological cure rate for cephapirin-treated cows
  - Clinical cure rate: N/A
  - Microbiological cure rate (at week 4 after treatment)
    - Untreated: 30% (8/27)
    - Cephapirin: 53% (10/19)
  - NNT for 1 additional cure: 5 (4.3)
  - Comments: treated cows had lower posttreatment SCC

A larger-scale clinical trial of IMM products for the treatment of clinical mastitis has been conducted in the United States within the past 5 years, and cephapirin was also included as a treatment in that trial.

- "Noninferiority Trial Comparing a First-Generation Cephalosporin with a Third-Generation Cephalosporin in the Treatment of Nonsevere Clinical Mastitis in Dairy Cows" by Schukken and colleagues[11]
  - Case definition: abnormal milk with or without signs of inflammation in the udder
    - Only 1 quarter affected with mastitis
    - No systemic signs of illness

- More than 25 days until scheduled to dry off
- No clinical mastitis within the last 30 days
  ○ Treatment groups
    ▪ Cephapirin 200 mg IMM every 12 hours × 2 doses
    ▪ Ceftiofur 125 mg IMM every 24 hours × 5 days
  ○ Cure definition
    ▪ Clinical: no clinical signs 10 and 17 days after treatment
    ▪ Microbiological: negative milk culture at 10 and 17 days after treatment
  ○ Treatment outcome differences: yes, ceftiofur had a significantly higher micro-biological cure rate for Gram-negative infections compared with cephapirin
  ○ Clinical cure rate: overall 62% (184/296)
    ▪ About 71% for cows with negative milk culture at enrollment
    ▪ About 63% for Gram-positive bacteria
    ▪ About 49% for Gram-negative bacteria
    ▪ Gram-positive pathogens: cephapirin 65%, ceftiofur 62%
    ▪ Gram-negative pathogens: cephapirin 50%, ceftiofur 44%
  ○ Microbiological cure rate: overall 67% (130/193)
    ▪ Cephapirin overall: 61% (59/96), Ceftiofur overall: 73% (71/97)
    ▪ Gram-positive pathogens: cephapirin 68%, ceftiofur 67%
    ▪ Gram-negative pathogens: cephapirin 50%, ceftiofur 79%
  ○ NNT for 1 additional cure: N/A no untreated controls

In summary, there is evidence that cephapirin improves the rate of microbiological cure of subclinical mastitis when compared with untreated controls and that it has comparable efficacy to ceftiofur for the resolution of clinical signs associated with mastitis caused by Gram-positive pathogens.

Ceftiofur

Ceftiofur (Spectramast LC; NADA 141-238) is a third-generation cephalosporin, so its spectrum of activity is expected to include more activity against Gram-negative pathogens than first-generation cephalosporins but less activity against Gram-positive species.

The product label states that Spectramast LC is indicated for the "treatment of clinical mastitis in lactating dairy cattle associated with coagulase-negative staphylococci, *Streptococcus dysgalactiae,* and *Escherichia coli.*" The FDA-approved dosing regimen is 1 tube containing 125 mg ceftiofur IMM every 24 hours for 2 to 8 total doses.[35]

A clinical trial done to test the efficacy of Spectramast LC before approval is published by the FDA.[36] The drug was evaluated at 2 dose levels; data for the approved tube dose of 125 mg cephapirin are reported here.

- "Freedom of Information Summary, Original New Animal Drug Application 141-238"[36]
  ○ Case definition: abnormal milk or signs of inflammation in the udder and positive CMT results
  ○ Treatment groups
    ▪ Untreated control
    ▪ Ceftiofur 62.5 mg IMM every 24 hours × 2 days
    ▪ Ceftiofur 125 mg IMM every 24 hours × 2 days
  ○ Cure definition
    ▪ Clinical: milk and udder returning to normal 14 days after the last treatment and remaining normal at 21 days posttreatment

- Microbiological: absence of the pretreatment pathogen at 14 and 21 days posttreatment
- Treatment outcome differences: yes, 125 mg ceftiofur had significantly higher clinical and microbiological cure rate than untreated controls.
- Clinical cure rate
  - Untreated controls: 64/117 (54.7%)
  - Ceftiofur 125 mg IMM 88/112 (78.6%)
- Microbiological cure rate: overall 67% (130/193)
  - Untreated controls: 41.3% (19/46)
  - Ceftiofur 125 mg: 70.4% (38/54)
- NNT for 1 additional cure at approved dose
  - Clinical: 5 (4.18)
  - Microbiological: 4 (3.44)

Ceftiofur has an FDA approval for varying durations of treatment; in 2004 Oliver and colleagues[37] published the results of a comparison of 3 different dosing regimens with no treatment of cases of subclinical mastitis:

- "Efficacy of Extended Ceftiofur Intramammary Therapy for Treatment of Subclinical Mastitis in Lactating Dairy Cows" by Oliver and colleagues[37]
  - Case definition: Initially screened using DHIA test greater than 400,000 cells/mL
    - Two milk cultures at 1-week interval, same pathogen isolated twice
  - Treatment groups
    - Untreated control
    - Ceftiofur 125 mg IMM every 24 hours × 2 days
    - Ceftiofur 125 mg IMM every 24 hours × 5 days
    - Ceftiofur 125 mg IMM every 24 hours × 8 days
  - Cure definition: negative milk culture 14 and 28 days after treatment
  - Treatment outcome differences: yes, all ceftiofur treated groups had more cures than untreated controls, and 8-day regimen had higher cure rate than 2-day regimen.
  - Microbiological cure rate: overall 67% (130/193)
    - Untreated control: 11% (4/38)
    - Ceftiofur × 2 days: 39% (19/49)
    - Ceftiofur × 5 days: 54% (22/41)
    - Ceftiofur × 8 days: 66% (25/38)
  - NNT for 1 additional cure
    - Two doses versus untreated control: 4 (3.6)
    - Eight doses versus 2 doses: 4 (3.7)
    - Eight doses versus untreated control: 2 (1.8)

Ceftiofur was also a treatment in the 2013 study[11] described in the section about cephapirin and in an earlier study that focused on Gram-negative pathogens:

- "Randomized Clinical Trial to Evaluate the Efficacy of a 5-Day Ceftiofur Hydrochloride Intramammary Treatment on Nonsevere Gram-negative Clinical Mastitis" by Schukken and colleagues[12]
  - Case criteria: abnormal milk with or without signs of inflammation in the udder
    - Only 1 quarter affected with mastitis (abnormal milk ± udder signs)
    - Microbial growth of coliform bacteria on culture with 24 hours of diagnosis
    - No systemic signs of illness
    - More than 25 days until scheduled to dry off

- No antimicrobial drug treatment within the last 14 days
- Treatment groups
  - Untreated controls
  - Ceftiofur 125 mg IMM every 24 hours × 5 days
- Cure definition
  - Clinical: no clinical signs 10 and 17 days after treatment
  - Microbiological: negative milk culture for pretreatment species and strain at 7 ± 2 and 14 ± 2 days after treatment
- Treatment outcome differences: yes, ceftiofur had significantly higher microbiological cure rate for *E coli* and *Klebsiella* spp but not *Enterobacter* spp
- Clinical cure rate: overall 50%
  - Cows missing both posttreatment evaluations (18 cows) classified as treatment failures
- Microbiological cure rate: overall 67% (130/193)
  - Untreated control: 38% (18/48)
  - Ceftiofur: 73% (41/56)
- NNT for 1 additional (microbiological) cure: 3 (2.85)
- Comments: Cows with less than 2 posttreatment cultures completed were classified as treatment failures. About 75% of untreated controls and 89% of treated cows had both samples completed; thus the rate of treatment failure in the untreated group may be inflated by cows for which posttreatment sampling was incomplete. For this reason, this study is excluded from summary tables. Cure rates varied substantially by farm (5 farms participated).

The studies regarding ceftiofur suggest that it is effective in improving cure rates of mastitis when compared with untreated controls and that 8 doses may have more efficacy than 2.

Macrolides: Pirlimycin

Pirlimycin

Pirlimycin (Pirsue, NADA 141-036) is a macrolide drug expected to have a spectrum of activity including Gram-positive mastitis pathogens.

Approved indications for the use of Pirsue are the "treatment of clinical and subclinical mastitis in lactating dairy cattle associated with *Staphylococcus* species such as *Staphylococcus aureus* and *Streptococcus* species such as *Streptococcus agalactiae*, *Streptococcus dysgalactiae*, and *Streptococcus uberis*." The label dose is 1 tube containing 50 mg of pirlimycin IMM every 24 hours up to 8 doses.[38]

- In a clinical trial[39] performed as part of the approval process, 3 dosing levels were evaluated; data are reported for the approved dose of 50 mg per treatment. The study did enroll cows with more than 1 infected quarter:
  - Case definition: abnormal milk ± udder inflammation
  - Treatment groups
    - Untreated control
    - Pirlimycin 50 mg IMM every 24 hours × 2 days
  - Cure definition (combined microbiological and clinical)
    - Negative results on milk culture 11 days after the first day of treatment and normal milk
  - Treatment outcome differences: yes
  - Cure rate (combined clinical and microbiological)
    - Untreated control: 28%
    - Pirlimycin 50 mg IMM every 24 hours × 2 days: 48%

- o NNT for 1 additional cure: 5
- o Note: "These clinical cases included staphylococcal and streptococcal isolates which include *S aureus, S agalactiae, S dysgalactiae*, and *S uberis*."

Other studies were published in the 2000s describing treatment of subclinical infection with pirlimycin; these studies are not reported here as they involved subclinical cases and enrolled cows with multiple infected quarters.

Based on the available evidence, it is reasonable to conclude that IMM therapy with pirlimycin does improve the likelihood of resolution of mastitis due to Gram-positive organisms when compared with untreated controls.

Summary

Prospective clinical trials evaluating IMM antimicrobial drug therapy for naturally occurring mastitis in dairy cows are not abundant. The studies that have been done have often found some degree of efficacy for IMM antimicrobial drug therapy in treating clinical mastitis in lactating dairy cows.

DRY COW THERAPY

IMM antimicrobial dry cow therapy (ADCT) formulations contain a long-acting antimicrobial drug and are infused into the mammary gland at the time of dry off. The purpose of ADCT is 2-fold: to treat any existing infections present at dry off and to prevent new infections that may be acquired during the dry period, thereby reducing the prevalence of IMI at calving. There are several benefits of ADCT compared with lactational therapy for IMI, including the following: a higher dose of antimicrobial drug is used; antimicrobial drug concentration is maintained in the udder for longer in the absence of regular milking, and the risk for violative milk residues may be reduced with proper use.[40] Antibiotic dry cow therapy has been shown to be highly effective at curing IMI. One meta-analysis of 22 studies published before 2003 on the effectiveness of ADCT estimated the cure risk for treated quarters was 78%, compared with a spontaneous cure risk of only 46%.[41]

Evidence-based decision making should be applied when selecting an appropriate ADCT formulation. As with products for lactating cows, most IMM ADCT products were introduced when contagious mastitis caused by *S aureus* and *S agalactiae* was a major concern for the dairy industry. Thus, most studies of the efficacy of these products were concerned primarily with these 2 pathogens. However, most subclinical infections present at dry off, as well as new infections acquired during the dry period, are likely caused by a broader mix of environmental pathogens, including environmental streptococci and coliforms. There is little evidence as to the efficacy of ADCT for these pathogens. The antimicrobials found in available ADCT products are the same as those found in lactating IMM products (**Table 5**), and therefore the expected spectra of activity are the same.

A study by Arruda and colleagues[42] comparing 3 commonly used ADCT formulations found no evidence of inferiority (no difference) between the 3 products in the following outcomes: prevalence of IMI at calving, cure of preexisting IMI, prevention of new IMI, risk for clinical mastitis up to 100 DIM, 305-day mature-equivalent milk production, linear somatic cell score, risk for the cow experiencing a clinical mastitis event, risk for culling or death, and risk for pregnancy by 100 DIM. These results suggest that, with regard to the 3 products studied, factors other than efficacy could be considered when choosing an ADCT product, such as cost, minimum dry period length, and milk and meat withholding times. Summary data from this and other studies are presented in **Table 6**. The studies presented are clinical trials of IMM

Table 5
Antimicrobial products approved in the United States for intramammary treatment of dry cows

Name (Active Compound)	Label Indication	Milk/Meat Withdrawal	Minimum Dry Period Length
ToMorrow/Cefa-Dri (300 mg cephapirin benzathine)	S agalactiae and S aureus, including penicillin-resistant strains	72 h milk/42 d meat	30 d
Spectramast DC (500 mg ceftiofur hydrochloride)	S aureus, S dysgalactiae, and S uberis	No milk/16 d meat	30 d
Quartermaster (1,000,000 IU procaine penicillin G and 1 g dihydrostreptomycin)	S aureus	96 h milk/60 d meat	42 d
Dry-Clox (500 mg cloxacillin benzathine)	Gram-positive bacteria including S agalactiae, penicillin-resistant and non–penicillinase-producing S aureus	No milk/30 d meat	30 d
Orbenin-DC (500 mg cloxacillin benzathine)	S agalactiae and S aureus	No milk/28 d meat	28 d
Albadry Plus (200,000 IU penicillin G procaine and 400 mg novobiocin sodium)	S aureus and S agalactiae	72 h milk/30 d meat	30 d
Go-Dry (100,000 IU penicillin G procaine)	S agalactiae	72 h milk/14 d meat	
Orbeseal (bismuth subnitrate; non-antimicrobial)	For the prevention of new IMI throughout the dry period	None	

Check treatment information and milk and meat withdrawal times with drug manufacturer before prescribing based on this information.

ADCT available in North America, with random allocation of cows (not heifers) to treatment groups (except where noted), with either a positive or negative control, and were published in English language journals. These studies span many years because of the dearth of more current studies. No attempt was made to correct for publication bias, whereby studies that showed a lower magnitude or no effect are less likely to be published. Rather, this is meant to be an overview of what is in fact a scant body of literature on the efficacy of ADCT formulations available in North America. This lack of evidence does not necessarily mean a lack of efficacy as the meta-analysis referenced earlier suggests. In addition, the pathogen distribution of infected quarters in these studies varies widely. Readers can assume that more current studies are more reflective of the pathogen distribution seen on today's dairies. Definitions of microbiological cure differed between studies, depending on how many samples were collected and at what interval, and whether or not the same or any pathogen had to be isolated from posttreatment samples to qualify as a cure failure.

Ceftiofur Hydrochloride

The product label for Spectramast DC (NADA 141-239) states that ceftiofur is "indicated for the treatment of subclinical mastitis in dairy cattle at the time of dry off associated with *Staphylococcus aureus*, *Streptococcus dysgalactiae*, and *Streptococcus uberis*." The FDA-approved dosing regimen is 1 tube containing 500 mg ceftiofur

Table 6
Summary of Intramammary antimicrobial dry cow therapy (ADCT) studies

Study	Treatment Comparisons	Microbiological Cure	NNT	New IMI	Comments
Arruda et al,[42] 2013 USA[a]	500 mg ceftiofur hydrochloride (1396 q[b])	88% (191/217)		11.9% (148/1239)	Noninferiority trial; no significant differences found
	300 mg cephapirin benzathine (1,476 q)	90% (252/281)		13.8% (187/1357)	
	10^6 IU procaine penicillin G and 1 g dihydrostreptomycin (1,492 q)	89% (216/243)		14.1% (192/1366)	
Hallberg et al,[44] 2005 USA[a]	500 mg ceftiofur (86 c[b])	61.8% (84/136); Greater than untreated control, P = .031	6.5	32.9% (71/216)[c]; Greater than untreated control, P = .029	Enrollment criteria: individual SCC≥400,000 cells/mL or LS ≥5; no CM at DO; no systemic or IMM treatment within 30 d of DO
	300 mg cephapirin benzathine (90 c)	56.3% (58/103)		36.4% (90/247)[c]	
	Untreated control (84 c)	46.4% (45/97)		46.7% (105/225)[c]	
Spectramast DC FDA Approval Study, 2005[45] USA[a,d]	500 mg ceftiofur hydrochloride	64.6% (115/178); P = .004 SA 44.4% (12/27) S dys 80% (12/15) S ub 83% (10/12)	5		583 Cows with SCC≥400,000 cells/ mL or an LS≥5 were enrolled
	Untreated control	45.0% (82/182) SA 20.7% (6/29) S dys 25% (2/8) S ub 62.5% (5/8)			

Study	Treatment	Cure rate		New IMI	Comments
Hogan et al,[47] 1994 USA[a,d]	300 mg cephapirin (186 c)	86.3% (182/211) SA 100% (20/20) CNS 78.2% (87/111) C bovis 98.4% (62/63) P<.05	3.8	Raw numbers not reported; ADCT reduced new IMI caused by environmental streptococci and C bovis (P<.05)	Only low SCC herds were enrolled (mean 215,000 cells/mL)
	Untreated control (93 c)	59.1% (140/237) SA 45% (20/44) CNS 62.7% (67/107) C bovis 63.9% (36/56)			
Cefa-Dri FDA Approval Study,[48] 1973 USA[a]	300 mg cephapirin benzathine (657 q)	86.5% (568/657)	4.3		All q in treatment and 65 q in control group were infected at dry off
	Untreated control (260 q)	63.1% (41/65)[e]			
Harmon et al,[49] 1986 USA[d]	300 mg cephapirin benzathine (151 q)	87.2% (34/39); P<.01	2.7	4.5% (5/112); P<.01	Results reported for minor pathogens only, including CNS and C bovis
	10⁶ IU procaine penicillin G and 1 g dihydrostreptomycin (132 q)	97.1% (33/34); P<.01	2.1	21.4% (21/98)	
	Untreated control (131 q)	50.0% (22/44)		18.4% (16/87)	
Cummins and McCaskey,[79] 1987 USA[a,d]	500 mg cloxacillin benzathine	73.6% (39/53)		28.6% (28/98)	Unclear if random assignment; no significant differences in cure or new IMI detected due to small n per group.
	Untreated control	51.0% (26/51)		31.5% (29/92)	
Pankey et al,[80] 1982a New Zealand[d]	500 mg cloxacillin benzathine	85.7% (90/105)			Cows not randomly allocated; results reported for SA, S ub, S ag only
	Untreated control	32.8% (20/61)			

(continued on next page)

Table 6
(continued)

Study	Treatment Comparisons	Microbiological Cure	NNT	New IMI	Comments
Browning et al,[81] 1990 Australia[a]	Not infected, not treated (350 c) Not infected, all q treated: 500 mg cloxacillin benzathine (350 c) Infected, infected q only treated: 500 mg cloxacillin benzathine (170 c) Infected, all q treated: 500 mg cloxacillin benzathine (170 c)	66% (182/275) 66% (181/275)		3.8% (54/1416) 2.1% (29/1384) 15.3% (62/405); P<.01 4.3% (18/421)	Low new IMI rate compared with other studies in North America
Shephard et al,[82] 2004 Australia[a]	500 mg cloxacillin benzathine (1174 c) 250 mg cephalonium (893 c)	70.7% (266/376) 80.3% (278/346); P = .02			
Bradley et al,[83] 2011 England[a]	150 mg cefquinome (161 c) 600 mg cloxacillin plus internal teat sealant (164 c) 600 mg cloxacillin alone (164 c)	84.6% (482/570) 89.7% (548/611) 82.2% (508/618)			Low SCC herds enrolled (BTSCC<250,000 cells/mL), cows with IMM or systemic treatment within 30 d previous to dry off were not enrolled
Rindsig et al,[53] 1978 USA[a]	Selective ADCT: 10[6] IU procaine penicillin G plus 1 g dihydrostreptomycin (112 c) Blanket ADCT: 10[6] IU procaine penicillin G plus 1 g dihydrostreptomycin (120 c)	88.2% (45/51) Treated 90.0% (36/40) Untreated 81.8% (9/11) 85.4% (41/48)		6.5% (29/448) 3.1% (15/480); P = .025	Alternate assignment to treatment groups. Selective DCT if SCC>500,000 cells/mL 1 m before dry off, or CMT score +2 or +3 at dry off, or history of CM in current lactation
Shultze et al,[54] 1983 USA[a]	10[6] IU procaine penicillin G plus 1 g dihydrostreptomycin (176/277 c infected 1 w before dry off) Untreated (4/143 c infected 1 w before dry off)	85.7% (108/126) SA 78% CNS 82% S spp. 88% Coli 87% 78.5% (51/65)			Not random allocation, cows with history of IMI selected for ADCT

Reference	Treatment group	Cure rate	Linear score	New IMI rate	Comments
Cook et al,[55] 2005 USA[a]	10^6 IU procaine penicillin G plus 1 g dihydrostreptomycin (1032 q)	80.6% (103/128)		16.5% (160/971)	Alternate enrollment
	10^6 IU procaine penicillin G plus 1 g dihydrostreptomycin, plus internal teat sealant (1080 q)	90.1% (114/127)		8.0% (81/1009); P = .08	
Albadry Plus FDA Approval Study, 2003[57] USA	200,000 IU procaine penicillin G and 400 mg novobiocin	SA 56%; S ag 78%; P<.002	SA 6.3; S ag 2.4		Total 1500 cows enrolled
	Untreated control	SA 40%, S ag 37%			
Pankey et al,[58] 1982b New Zealand[d]	200,000 IU procaine penicillin G and 400 mg novobiocin (min 40 c)	61.3% (38/62); P<.05	5.4	7.3% (18/248)	Cure results reported for SA only; for new IMI SA, S ub only
	Untreated controls (min 40 c)	41.2% (21/50)		11.7% (27/230)	
Heald et al,[59] 1977 USA[d]	200,000 IU procaine penicillin G and 400 mg novobiocin (107 q)	88.5% (23/26)	4.9	15.9%	Sequential assignment to 9 treatment groups, producer allowed to reassign cows to receive ADCT; results reported for GP only
	Untreated controls (100 q)	67.9% (19/28)		14.0%	

Abbreviations: BTSCC, bulk tank SCC; CM, clinical mastitis; CNS, coagulase negative staphylococci; Coli, coliforms; DO, dry off; GP, Gram-positive pathogens; LS, linear score; SA, S aureus; S ag, S agalactiae; S dys, S dysgalactiae; S spp, Streptococcus species; S ub, S uberis.
[a] Results reported for all naturally occurring pathogens.
[b] When available, number assigned in each treatment group (c = cow, q = quarter).
[c] Recalculated as follows: 1-Prevention success rate (# infected quarters postcalving/# uninfected quarters at dry off).
[d] Some treatment groups omitted because not available in North America, or nonantimicrobial.
[e] Recalculated using only cows infected at dry off as denominator.
Data from Refs.[42,44,45,47–49,53–55,57–59,78–83]

into each affected quarter at the time of dry off, no later than 30 days before calving.[43] Spectramast DC was approved for use in 2005, and thus the few studies that include ceftiofur hydrochloride as a treatment are more current and may be more generalizable to modern dairy farms in North America. Estimated overall microbiological cure risk ranges from 62% to 88%, with new IMI risk between 12% and 22%. The 2 studies that included a negative control group allowed calculation of an NNT (5 or 6.5), meaning 5 or 6.5 treatments are needed to affect 1 cure.[43–45]

Cephapirin Benzathine

The product label for ToMorrow (NADA 108-114) states that cephapirin is indicated for the treatment of any dry cow known to harbor the following organisms in the udder at dry off: S agalactiae and S aureus, including penicillin-resistant strains. The FDA-approved dosing regimen is 1 tube containing 300 mg cephapirin infused into each quarter at the time of dry off, to be used no later than 30 days before calving.[46] Three of the studies selected showed a microbiological cure risk for cephapirin treatment as 86% to 87%, with one smaller study reporting a cure risk of only 56%. The NNT from the larger studies was 2.7 to 4.3. New IMI was not consistently reported, but in one study cephapirin ADCT was found to significantly reduce IMI caused by environmental streptococci and Corynebacterium bovis, and in another, the drug significantly reduced IMI caused by minor pathogens including coagulase-negative staphylococci and C bovis.[43,45,47–49]

Cloxacillin Benzathine

The product label for Dry-Clox (NADA 055-058) states that cloxacillin is indicated for the treatment of any dry cow known to harbor susceptible organisms in the udder at dry off, "or which has had repeated attacks of mastitis during the previous lactation, or is affected with mastitis at drying off, if caused by susceptible organisms." Organisms with demonstrated susceptibility are S agalactiae and S aureus, including penicillin-resistant strains. The FDA-approved dosing regimen is 1 tube containing 500 mg cloxacillin benzathine infused into each quarter at the time of dry off. This product must be used no later than 30 days before calving.[50] The product label for Orbenin-DC (NADA 55-069) is similar.[51] Microbiological cure risk for cloxacillin ADCT ranged from 66% to 82%. The highest cure rates were achieved with a product that contains 600 mg cloxacillin, which is 100 mg more than what is currently available in North America. Of the 2 cloxacillin studies with a negative control group, 1 was not powered to detect a significant difference and 1 did not have random allocation to treatment groups. Thus, the calculation of NNT from these studies is not advisable. Although many studies exist that use cloxacillin as a positive control to compare with other IMM formulations, there is little high-quality evidence for efficacy of cloxacillin compared with a negative control.

Procaine Penicillin G

Go-Dry (NDC10515-012-10) is indicated for udder infections caused by S agalactiae, for use at dry off. One tube contains 100,000 IU procaine penicillin G. No studies were found for this dose of procaine penicillin.

Procaine Penicillin G and Dihydrostreptomycin

Quartermaster (NADA 055-028) is indicated "for intramammary use to reduce the frequency of existing infection and to prevent new infections with Staphylococcus aureus in dry cows." The FDA-approved dosing regimen is 1 tube containing 1,000,000 IU procaine penicillin G and 1 g dihydrostreptomycin infused into each quarter at the time of dry off and no later than 6 weeks before calving.[52] Reported microbiological cure rates for procaine penicillin G plus dihydrostreptomycin ADCT are high (81%–90%); however, only 1 study with a negative control group was found (97.1%, minor pathogens only considered). The most recent study conducted by Arruda and colleagues reported a cure risk of 89% and a new IMI risk of 14.1%.[42] Some of the available studies compared blanket ADCT to selective ADCT with this formulation, which may provide some insight into expected cure rates but does not allow calculation of NNT. The NNT calculated (2.1) for the 1 negative controlled study would only apply to minor pathogens, including coagulase-negative staphylococci and C bovis.[43,50,53–55]

Procaine Penicillin G and Novobiocin Sodium

The product label for Albadry Plus (NADA 55-098) states that procaine penicillin G and novobiocin sodium are indicated for "the treatment, in dry cows only, of subclinical mastitis caused by susceptible strains of Staphylococcus aureus and Streptococcus agalactiae." The FDA-approved dosing regimen is 1 tube containing 200,000 IU procaine penicillin G and 400 mg novobiocin sodium infused into each quarter at the time of dry off and no later than 30 days before calving.[56] The studies included here only reported cure and new IMI risk for Gram-positive pathogens. Microbiological cure rates ranged from 56% and 61% for S aureus to 89% for all Gram-positive pathogens combined. NNT for S aureus was 5.4 and 6.3. The NNT for all Gram-positive pathogens combined was 4.9.[57–59]

Although ADCT is generally considered effective at curing existing infection, there is less evidence for efficacy in preventing new infections, particularly during the high-risk prepartum period when the concentration of ADCT in the mammary gland is significantly reduced. Various studies have estimated the proportion of quarters developing new IMI during the dry period to be between 8% and 25%.[60,61] Internal teat sealants are often used as an adjunct therapy to help further reduce the risk of new infection during the dry period. Internal teat sealants contain a nonantimicrobial, inert substance (bismuth subnitrate) that is insoluble in milk and when infused correctly into the teat persist as an internal barrier against infection throughout the dry period. A meta-analysis assessed the evidence for efficacy of an internal teat sealant when used alone or in combination with ADCT. This study found that the use of an internal teat sealant (alone or in combination with ADCT) significantly reduced the risk of IMI and clinical mastitis in lactating cows (**Table 7**).[62] However, estimates of effect differed between studies that used an internal teat sealant in combination with ADCT and

Table 7
Relative risk of IMI and clinical mastitis in dairy cows treated with internal teat sealant alone or in presence of intramammary antimicrobial dry cow therapy and number needed to treat

Outcome	Subgroup (Number of Comparisons)	Relative Risk (95% Confidence Interval)	P-Value	NNT
IMI	Positive control[a] (n = 13)	0.75 (0.67, 0.83)	<.001	20
	Negative control[b] (n = 4)	0.27 (0.13, 0.55)	<.001	7
Clinical mastitis	Positive control (n = 14)	0.71 (0.62, 0.82)	<.001	21
	Negative control (n = 7)	0.52 (0.37, 0.75)	<.001	13

[a] Positive control: comparison with ADCT alone.
[b] Negative control: comparison with no treatment.
From Rabiee AR, Lean, IJ. The effect of internal teat sealant products (Teatseal and Orbeseal) on intramammary infection, clinical mastitis, and somatic cell counts in lactating dairy cows: a meta-analysis. J Dairy Sci 2013;96(11):6921.

those that used internal teat sealant alone. The investigators of that study suggest that the estimate of efficacy used be specific to whether internal teat sealant is used alone or in combination. Many of the studies that used teat sealant alone used SCC criteria to select for treatment cows presumed to be uninfected.

Other therapeutic methods that have been considered to decrease IMI at calving include treating prepartum heifers and treating dry cows with a lactational IMM formulation prepartum. Although these practices have been shown to be effective at reducing the prevalence of IMI at calving, little evidence exists to support widespread adoption of these practices, particularly as to the economic and practical feasibility, except possibly in cases in which risk of infection is high and other management strategies are not possible or are ineffective.[63,64] Nontherapeutic strategies are also important and include vaccination, nutrition, dry off strategy, and management of environmental hygiene.

Although the blanket application of ADCT is common in North America (72.3% of US dairy operations[64]), the selective application of ADCT is the focus of much current research; this is driven in large part by regulations in some European countries that preclude the use of antimicrobials for prevention of disease. These studies aim primarily to develop and evaluate selection criteria to be used on the farm to determine which cows should be treated with ADCT and/or an internal teat sealant. With the prevalence of IMI at dry off estimated at 13% to 35% in North American studies,[65–67] the ability to select only infected cows for ADCT would result in a significant decrease in the use of antimicrobials. In addition, the use of an internal teat sealant provides an effective, nonantimicrobial option for prevention of new infection. Selection criteria that have been evaluated include SCC and clinical mastitis history before dry off,[67,68] the CMT,[69] and the 3M Aerobic Count Petrifilm (3M Canada, London, Ontario) on-farm culture system.[70,71] Although recent studies have demonstrated that selection for ADCT at the cow level (all quarters of an infected cow are treated with ADCT) can be as effective as blanket ADCT when an internal teat sealant is used,[72] more work is needed to determine whether quarter-level selective ADCT is effective and to identify the optimal selection criteria and ADCT strategy for herds in North America.

Much research has also been focused on systemic administration of antimicrobials at dry off.[73–75] However, no systemic antimicrobial products are labeled for this use in the United States. Following the Animal Medicinal Drug Use Clarification Act and given that there are IMM products labeled and effective for the elimination of IMI at dry off, the authors feel that systemic antimicrobial use at dry off is not justifiable without clear evidence that the available IMM products are not likely to be clinically effective in a given situation.

SUMMARY AND DISCUSSION

Although much of the evidence for efficacy of IMM antimicrobial treatments for mastitis is dated, especially in regard to the distribution of mastitis pathogens found on dairies, one can draw some conclusions based on presumed spectra of activity and available clinical trial data. The expected spectrum of activity and in vitro pathogen susceptibility to a particular antimicrobial drug may not be correlated with efficacy in the mammary gland. Many of the available IMM formations have demonstrated efficacy against Gram-positive pathogens. There is less evidence to support efficacy against Gram-negative pathogens for many of the formulations currently available in North America. Differences in efficacy between Gram-positive and Gram-negative pathogens may be due to several factors, including mode of action of the drug, pathogen virulence, and spontaneous cure rates. Based on spectrum of activity and clinical trial data, there is evidence that ceftiofur hydrochloride has improved efficacy against Gram-negative pathogens. In contrast, pirlimycin hydro-chloride is known be ineffective against Gram-negative pathogens, based primarily on expected spectrum of activity, but does have demonstrated efficacy against Gram-positive pathogens. Other than these differences, there is little evidence to sug-gest that the choice of one antimicrobial drug may result in significantly better out-comes than another antimicrobial drug.

The NNT is a useful number to demonstrate that utility of a treatment depends both on the number of cures in the treatment group and on the rate of spontaneous cures in the untreated control group. In cases in which the spontaneous cure rate is likely to be high, as in cases caused by E coli,[3,25,26] the NNT may be large even if the cure rate for treated cows is high. In cases in which the spontaneous cure rate is likely to be low, the NNT may be lower even if the cure rate in the treatment group is only moderate. The NNT is also useful to help assess the economic implications of treatment. When NNT is low, the treatment cost per favorable outcome is low, compared with when the NNT is high.

However, the specific pathogen causing infection, the chronicity of infection, and the immune status of the cow likely have a greater influence on the case outcome than the choice of antimicrobial drug. For a review of estimated spontaneous and treatment cure rates by pathogen, see article by Pinzón-Sánchez and colleagues.[6] It is also likely that there are significant variations in success rates depending on the strain of the pathogen species and other factors that are farm-dependent. For example, some dairies have higher cure rates for a particular pathogen than other dairies. Other practical factors that must be considered include differences in cost, treatment regimen (particularly duration of therapy and once-a-day vs every 12-hour dosing), and milk and meat withholding times. It is logical to assume that extended duration therapy results in greater treatment success rates, and this has been demon-strated in the literature.[76,77] However, only 2 lactational IMM antimicrobial products are labeled for extended duration therapy, and factors such as cost and degree of improvement in cure rates (NNT) should be considered. Pinzón-Sánchez and col-leagues[6] estimated that for mild or moderate clinical mastitis, short-duration (2-day) therapy for Gram-positive pathogens and no antimicrobial therapy for Gram-negative pathogens or in cases in which no pathogen is recovered is the economically optimal strategy.

To achieve maximum treatment success rates, only cases of clinical mastitis that are likely to benefit should receive IMM antimicrobial therapy. Cows with a strong indi-cation of chronic IMI, or with concurrent disease, should perhaps be managed in other ways. Lastly, it is important to monitor treatment success rates to ensure that appro-priate farm-specific protocols are in place. The pathogen profile in a particular dairy may change between seasons, when new cows are added to the herd, or simply as a result of mastitis control strategies. Monitoring bulk tank and clinical mastitis cul-tures concurrently with treatment outcomes can help producers and practitioners make adjustments to maximize success. Practitioners must also always consider the potential for violative residues with the use of antimicrobial drugs for mastitis and should make every effort to minimize this risk by adhering to label use and ensuring protocol compliance by everyone involved in mastitis treatment on dairies.

REFERENCES

1. Leslie KE, Petersson-Wolfe CS. Assessment and management of pain in dairy cows with clinical mastitis. Vet Clin North Am 2012;28(2):289–305.

2. Hallén Sandgren C, Persson Waller K, Emanuelson U. Therapeutic effects of systemic or intramammary antimicrobial treatment of bovine subclinical mastitis during lactation. Vet J 2008;175:108–17.

3. Wilson DJ, Gonzalez RN, Case KL, et al. Comparison of seven antibiotic treatments with no treatment for bacteriological efficacy against bovine mastitis pathogens. J Dairy Sci 1999;82(8):1664–70.

4. McDermott MP, Erb HN, Natzke RP, et al. Cost benefit analysis of lactation therapy with somatic cell counts as indications for treatment. J Dairy Sci 1983;66:1198–203.

5. Pinzón-Sánchez C, Ruegg PL. Risk factors associated with short-term post-treatment outcomes of clinical mastitis. J Dairy Sci 2011;94(7):3397–410.

6. Pinzón-Sánchez C, Cabrera VE, Ruegg PL. Decision tree analysis of treatment strategies for mild and moderate cases of clinical mastitis occurring in early lactation. J Dairy Sci 2011;94(4):1873–92.

7. Fox LK. Mycoplasma mastitis: causes, transmission, and control. Vet Clin North Am Food Anim Pract 2012;28(2):225–37.

8. Oliver SP, Mitchell BA. Prevalence of mastitis pathogens in herds participating in a mastitis control program. J Dairy Sci 1984;67(10):2436–40.

9. González RN, Jasper DE, Farver TB, et al. Prevalence of udder infections and mastitis in 50 California dairy herds. J Am Vet Med Assoc 1988;193(3):323.

10. Lago A, Godden SM, Bey R, et al. The selective treatment of clinical mastitis based on on-farm culture results: I. Effects on antibiotic use, milk withholding time, and short-term clinical and bacteriological outcomes. J Dairy Sci 2011;94(9):4441–56.

11. Schukken YH, Zurakowski MJ, Rauch BJ, et al. Noninferiority trial comparing a first-generation cephalosporin with a third-generation cephalosporin in the treatment of nonsevere clinical mastitis in dairy cows. J Dairy Sci 2013;96(10):6763–74.

12. Schukken YH, Bennett GJ, Zurakowski MJ, et al. Randomized clinical trial to evaluate the efficacy of a 5-day ceftiofur hydrochloride intramammary treatment on nonsevere gram-negative clinical mastitis. J Dairy Sci 2011;94(12):6203–15.

13. Pol M, Ruegg PL. Relationship between antimicrobial drug usage and antimicrobial susceptibility of gram-positive mastitis pathogens. J Dairy Sci 2007;90:262–73.

14. Bradley AJ, Green MJ. Factors affecting cure when treating bovine clinical mastitis with cephalosporin-based intramammary preparations. J Dairy Sci 2009;92(5):1941–53.

15. Constable PD, Morin DE. Use of antimicrobial susceptibility testing of bacterial pathogens isolated from the milk of dairy cows with clinical mastitis to predict response to treatment with cephapirin and oxytetracycline. J Am Vet Med Assoc 2002;221(1):103–8.

16. Sol J, Sampimon OC, Barkema HW, et al. Factors associated with cure after therapy of clinical mastitis caused by Staphylococcus aureus. J Dairy Sci 2000;83:278–84.

17. Sol J, Sampimon OC, Snoep JJ, et al. Factors associated with bacteriological cure after dry cow treatment of subclinical Staphylococcus aureus mastitis with antibiotics. J Dairy Sci 1994;77:75–9.

18. Sol J, Sampimon OC, Snoep JJ, et al. Factors associated with bacteriological cure during lactation after therapy for subclinical mastitis caused by Staphylococcus aureus. J Dairy Sci 1997;80:2803–8.

19. Barkema HW, Schukken YH, Zadoks RN. Invited review: the role of cow, pathogen, and treatment regimen in the therapeutic success of bovine Staphylococcus aureus mastitis. J Dairy Sci 2006;89(6):1877–95.

20. Deluyker HA, Van Oye SN, Boucher JF, et al. Factors affecting cure and somatic cell count after pirlimycin treatment of subclinical mastitis in lactating cows. J Dairy Sci 2005;88(2):604–14.

21. Rossitto PV, Ruiz L, Kikuchi Y, et al. Antibiotic susceptibility patterns for environmental streptococci isolated from bovine mastitis in central California dairies. J Dairy Sci 2002;85(1):132–8.

22. Hoe FG, Ruegg PL. Relationship between antimicrobial susceptibility of clinical mastitis pathogens and treatment outcome in cows. J Am Vet Med Assoc 2005;227(9):1461–8.

23. Bartlett PC, Miller GY, Lance SE, et al. Clinical mastitis and intramammary infections on Ohio dairy farms. Prev Vet Med 1992;12:59–71.

24. Olde Riekerink R, Barkema H, Poole D, et al. Risk factors for incidence rate of clinical mastitis in a nationwide study on Canadian dairy farms. In: Proceedings of the 46th Annual Meeting of the National Mastitis Council. San Antonio (TX): National Mastitis Council, Madison, WI, 2008. p. 204.

25. Guterbock WM, Van Eenennaam AL, Anderson RJ, et al. Efficacy of intramammary antibiotic therapy for treatment of clinical mastitis caused by environmental pathogens. J Dairy Sci 1993;76:3437–44.

26. Morin DE, Shanks RD, McCoy GC. Comparison of antibiotic administration in conjunction with supportive measures versus supportive measures alone for treatment of dairy cows with clinical mastitis. J Am Vet Med Assoc 1998;213:676–84.

27. Amoxi-Mast prescribing information. Available at: http://www.merck-animal-health-usa.com/binaries/Amoxi-Mastitis_Tubes_tcm96-85711.pdf. Accessed October 10, 2014.

28. Freedom of Information Summary; NADA 055-100, US Food and Drug Administration.

29. Roberson JR, Warnick LD, Moore G. Mild to moderate clinical mastitis: efficacy of intramammary amoxicillin, frequent milk-out, a combined intramammary amoxicillin, and frequent milk-out treatment versus no treatment. J Dairy Sci 2004; 87(3):583–92.

30. Hetacin-K prescribing information. Available at: http://www.bi-vetmedica.com/content/dam/internet/ah/vetmedica/com_EN/product_files/hetacin-k/Hetacin-K%20Pkg%20Insert.pdf. Accessed October 10, 2014.

31. Dariclox prescribing information. Available at: http://www.merck-animal-health-usa.com/binaries/Amoxi-Mastitis_Tubes_tcm96-85711.pdf. Accessed October 10, 2014.

32. Shephard RW, Malmo J, Pfeiffer DU. A clinical trial to evaluate the effectiveness of antibiotic treatment of lactating cows with high somatic cell counts in their milk. Aust Vet J 2000;78(11):763–8.

33. ToDay prescribing information. Available at: http://www.bi-vetmedica.com/main/cattle/ToDay.html. Accessed October 10, 2014.

34. Rosenberg JB, Love B, Patterson DL. Bacterial cure and somatic cell count response of dairy cows with a positive California mastitis test at calving to therapy with cephapirin sodium. Vet Ther 2002;3(4):381.

35. Spectramast LC prescribing information. Available at: https://www.zoetisus.com/products/dairy/spectramast-lc-_ceftiofur-hydrochloride_-sterile-suspension.aspx. Accessed October 10, 2014.

36. Freedom of information summary; NADA 141–238: SPECTRAMAST LC sterile suspension (ceftiofur hydrochloride) US Food and Drug Administration (2005). Available at: http://www.fda.gov/downloads/AnimalVeterinary/Products/ApprovedAnimalDrugProducts/FOIADrugSummaries/ucm118051.pdf. Accessed November 21, 2014.

37. Oliver SP, Gillespie BE, Headrick SJ, et al. Efficacy of extended ceftiofur intra-mammary therapy for treatment of subclinical mastitis in lactating dairy cows. J Dairy Sci 2004;87(8):2393–400.

38. Pirsue prescribing information. Available at: https://www.zoetisus.com/_locale-assets/mcm-portal-assets/products/pdf/pirsue.pdf. Accessed October 10, 2014.

39. Freedom of information summary; NADA 141–036: PIRSUE sterile solution (pirlimycin hydrochloride). US Food and Drug Administration (2007). Available at: http://www.fda.gov/downloads/AnimalVeterinary/Products/ApprovedAnimalDrug Products/FOIADrugSummaries/ucm116138.pdf. Accessed November 21, 2014.

40. Cameron M, Keefe G. Dry cow management. In: Proceedings of the 2014 Regional Meeting of the National Mastitis Council. Ghent, Belgium: National Mastitis Council, Madison, WI, 2014. p. 36.

41. Halasa T, Østerås O, Hogeveen H, et al. Meta-analysis of dry cow management for dairy cattle. Part 1. Protection against new intramammary infections. J Dairy Sci 2009;92:3134–49.

42. Arruda AG, Godden S, Rapnicki P, et al. Randomized noninferiority clinical trial evaluating 3 commercial dry cow mastitis preparations: I. Quarter-level outcomes. J Dairy Sci 2013;96:6390–9.

43. Spectramast DC prescribing information. Available at: https://www.zoetisus.com/products/dairy/spectramast-dc.aspx. Accessed October 11, 2014.

44. Hallberg JW, Wachowski M, Moseley WM, et al. Efficacy of intramammary infusion of ceftiofur hydrochloride at drying off for treatment and prevention of bovine mastitis during the nonlactating period. Vet Ther 2005;7(1):35–42.

45. Freedom of information summary; NADA 141–239: SPECTRAMAST DC sterile sus-pension (ceftiofur hydrochloride), US Food and Drug Administration. 2005. Available at: http://www.fda.gov/downloads/AnimalVeterinary/Products/ApprovedAnimalDrug Products/FOIADrugSummaries/ucm118055.pdf. Accessed November 21, 2014.

46. ToMorrow Prescribing Information. Available at: http://www.bi-vetmedica.com/main/cattle/ToMorrow.html. Accessed October 11, 2014.

47. Hogan JS, Smith KL, Todhunter DA, et al. Efficacy of dry cow therapy and a *Propionibacterium acnes* product in herds with low somatic cell count. J Dairy Sci 1994;77(11):3331–7.

48. Freedom of information summary; NADA 108–114: Cefa-Dri; ToMorrow Infusion; US Food and Drug Administration (1973).

49. Harmon RJ, Crist WL, Hemken RW, et al. Prevalence of minor udder pathogens after intramammary dry treatment. J Dairy Sci 1986;69(3):843–9.

50. Dry-Clox prescribing information. Available at: http://www.bi-vetmedica.com/main/cattle/dry-clox.html. Accessed October 11, 2014.

51. Orbenin-DC prescribing information. Available at: http://www.merck-animal-health-usa.com/products/130_163357/productdetails_130_163721.aspx. Accessed October 11, 2014.

52. Quartermaster prescribing information. Available at: http://www.drugs.com/vet/quartermaster.html. Accessed October 11, 2014.

53. Rindsig RB, Rodewald RG, Smith AR, et al. Complete versus selective dry cow therapy for mastitis control. J Dairy Sci 1978;61(10):1483–97.

54. Schultze WD. Effects of a selective regimen of dry cow therapy on intramammary infection and on antibiotic sensitivity of surviving pathogens. J Dairy Sci 1983;66(4):892–903.

55. Cook NB, Pionek D, Sharp P. An assessment of the benefits of Orbeseal when used in combination with dry cow antibiotic therapy in three commercial dairy herds. Bov Pract 2005;39:83–94.

56. Albadry Plus prescribing information. Available at: https://www.zoetisus.com/products/dairy/albadry-plus-suspension.aspx. Accessed October 11, 2014.
57. Freedom of information summary; NADA 055–098: Albadry plus suspension, US Food and Drug Administration (2003).
58. Pankey JW, Barker RM, Twomey A, et al. Comparative efficacy of dry-cow treatment regimens against *Staphylococcus aureus*. N Z Vet J 1982;30(1–2):13–5.
59. Heald CW, Jones GM, Nickerson S, et al. Mastitis control by penicillin and novobiocin at drying-off. Can Vet J 1977;18(7):171–80.
60. Eberhart RJ. Management of dry cows to reduce mastitis. J Dairy Sci 1986;69: 1721–32.
61. Godden S, Rapnicki P, Stewart S, et al. Effectiveness of an internal teat seal in the prevention of new intramammary infections during the dry and early-lactation periods in dairy cows when used with a dry cow intramammary antibiotic. J Dairy Sci 2003;86:3899–911.
62. Rabiee AR, Lean IJ. The effect of internal teat sealant products (Teatseal and Orbeseal) on intramammary infection, clinical mastitis, and somatic cell counts in lactating dairy cows: a meta-analysis. J Dairy Sci 2013;96(11):6915–31.
63. De Vliegher S, Fox LK, Piepers S, et al. Invited review: mastitis in dairy heifers: nature of the disease, potential impact, prevention, and control. J Dairy Sci 2012;95(3):1025–40.
64. USDA-NAHMS (US Department of Agriculture National Animal Health Monitoring System). 2008. Dairy 2007. Part III: Reference of dairy cattle health and management practices in the United States, 2007. Available at: http://www.aphis.usda.gov/animal_health/nahms/dairy/downloads/dairy07/Dairy07_dr_PartIII_rev.pdf. Accessed October 6, 2014.
65. Oliver SP, Mitchell BA. Susceptibility of bovine mammary gland to infections during the dry period. J Dairy Sci 1983;66:1162–6.
66. Pantoja JC, Hulland C, Ruegg PL. Dynamics of somatic cell counts and intramammary infections across the dry period. Prev Vet Med 2009;90:43–54.
67. Torres AH, Rajala-Schultz PJ, Degraves FJ, et al. Using dairy herd improvement records and clinical mastitis history to identify subclinical mastitis infections at dry-off. J Dairy Res 2008;75:240–7.
68. Rajala-Schultz PJ, Torres AH, Degraves FJ. Milk yield and somatic cell count during the following lactation after selective treatment of cows at dry-off. J Dairy Res 2011;78:489–99.
69. Sanford CJ, Keefe GP, Sanchez J, et al. Test characteristics from latent-class models of the California mastitis test. Prev Vet Med 2006;77:96–108.
70. Cameron M, Keefe GP, Roy JP, et al. Evaluation of a 3M Petrifilm on-farm culture system for the detection of intramammary infection at the end of lactation. Prev Vet Med 2013;111:1–9.
71. Cameron M, McKenna SL, MacDonald KA, et al. Evaluation of selective dry cow treatment following on-farm culture: risk of postcalving intramammary infection and clinical mastitis in the subsequent lactation. J Dairy Sci 2014; 97(1):270–84.
72. Hockett, M., and R. Rodriguez. 2013. Evaluation of milk leucocyte differential diagnosis for selective dry cow therapy. J Anim Sci Vol. 91, E-Suppl. 2/J Dairy Sci Vol. 96, E-Suppl. 1. pp 384.
73. Ataee O, Hovareshti P, Bolourchi M, et al. Effect of systemic antibacterial administration during prepartum period on coagulase negative staphylococcal intramammary infection in Holstein heifers. Iranian J Vet Research 2009;10(3): 255–9.

74. Bolourchi M, Hovareshti P, Tabatabayi AH. Comparison of the effects of local and systemic dry cow therapy for staphylococcal mastitis control. Prev Vet Med 1996;25(1):63–7.

75. Erskine RJ, Bartlett PC, Crawshaw PC, et al. Efficacy of intramuscular oxytetracycline as a dry cow treatment for *Staphylococcus aureus* mastitis. J Dairy Sci 1994;77:3347–53.

76. Oliver SP, Almeida RA, Gillespie BE, et al. Extended ceftiofur therapy for treatment of experimentally induced *Streptococcus uberis* mastitis in lactating dairy cattle. J Dairy Sci 2004;87:3322–9.

77. Gillespie BE, Moorehead H, Lunn P, et al. Efficacy of extended pirlimycin hydrochloride therapy for treatment of environmental Streptococcus spp. and Staphylococcus aureus intramammary infections in lactating dairy cows. Vet Ther 2002;3(4):373–80.

78. Freedom of information summary; NADA 108–114, Cefa-Dri (cephapirin benzathine) for intramammary infusion into dry cows.

79. Cummins KA, McCaskey TA. Multiple infusions of cloxacillin for treatment of mastitis during the dry period. Journal of dairy science 1987;70(12):2658–65.

80. Pankey JW, Barker RM, Twomey A, et al. A note on effectiveness of dry cow therapy in New Zealand dairy herds. New Zealand veterinary journal 1982;30(4):50–2.

81. Browning JW, Mein GA, Barton M. Effects of antibiotic therapy at drying off on mastitis in the dry period and early lactation. Australian veterinary journal 1990;67(12):440–2.

82. Shephard RW, Burman S, Marcun P. A comparative field trial of cephalonium and cloxacillin for dry cow therapy for mastitis in Australian dairy cows. Australian veterinary journal 2004;82(10):624–9.

83. Bradley AJ, Breen JE, Payne B, et al. A comparison of broad-spectrum and narrow-spectrum dry cow therapy used alone and in combination with a teat sealant. Journal of dairy science 2011;94(2):692–704.

Antimicrobial Decision Making for Enteric Diseases of Cattle

Geof Smith, DVM, MS, PhD

KEYWORDS

- Antimicrobials • Calf diarrhea • Diarrhea • Pharmacology • *Salmonella*

KEY POINTS

- In general, most enteric diseases of adult cattle would not likely benefit from antimicrobial therapy unless *Salmonella* is suspected.
- Based on current research, the feeding of oral antibiotics to calves to prevent diarrhea cannot be recommended.
- The use of certain antimicrobials to treat select cases of calf diarrhea may be effective in reducing mortality and decreasing the severity and duration of diarrhea; unfortunately, it is unlikely that any of the antibiotics that are currently approved for the treatment of diarrhea in the United States would be effective.
- Instead of mass medicating large numbers of calves, antimicrobial therapy should be targeted to specific animals that are likely to develop septicemia or have systemic signs of disease.

Diarrhea is the leading cause of calf mortality before weaning in both beef and dairy calves. Therefore, both veterinarians and producers should put some effort into designing rational and efficacious protocols for both prevention and treatment of diarrhea. Antimicrobials have long been used to prevent calf diarrhea and are often administered as a treatment. However, it is important to prevent unnecessary use of antibiotics in food animal species to limit the development of resistant bacteria. Enteric diseases are also common in adult cattle, and both beef and dairy practitioners are often asked to create treatment protocols for diarrhea. As diagnostic testing is often not available, these protocols are generally based on knowledge of the most likely pathogen and the veterinarian's clinical experience. This article reviews existing data on antibiotics given to both calves and adult cattle for the prevention and/or treatment of enteric disease. Based on current research, the administration of oral

The author has nothing to disclose.
Department of Population Health & Pathobiology, North Carolina State University, 1060 William Moore Drive, Raleigh, NC 27607, USA
E-mail address: Geoffrey_Smith@ncsu.edu

antibiotics to calves to prevent diarrhea cannot be recommended. However, the use of certain antimicrobials to treat select cases of calf diarrhea may be effective in reducing mortality and decreasing the severity and duration of diarrhea. Unfortunately, it is unlikely that any of the antibiotics that are currently approved for the treatment of diarrhea in the United States would be effective. Instead of mass medicating large numbers of animals, antimicrobial therapy should be targeted to specific animals that are likely to develop septicemia or have systemic signs of disease.

ENTERIC DISEASES OF ADULT CATTLE

There are many causes of diarrhea in adult cattle, and the vast majority of these do not warrant antimicrobial therapy. Common enteric diseases of cattle include simple indigestion, rumen acidosis, parasites, coccidiosis, bovine viral diarrhea (BVD), winter dysentery, Salmonella, paratuberculosis (Johne disease), molybdenosis (copper deficiency), and malignant catarrhal fever (MCF), along with a wide range of toxicities including a host of poisonous plants. The only disease on this list that is likely to truly benefit from antimicrobial therapy is Salmonella enteritis; however, an argument could be made for BVD and MCF. Both these diseases suppress normal immune function and can lead to an increased occurrence of secondary bacterial infections. It is well understood that BVD is associated with the bovine respiratory disease complex and can lead to higher rates of bacterial pneumonia.[1] However, cases of severe Salmonella enteritis have also been reported after BVD infection in cattle causing significant mortality.[2] Therefore, it would not be inappropriate to administer a broad-spectrum antimicrobial to cattle suspected of having BVD or MCF, likely one that is labeled for metaphylactic use in cattle at high risk for developing respiratory disease.

It is also important to note that many toxic cows with severe mastitis, metritis, or peritonitis often have diarrhea that is a direct result of endotoxemia.[3] The mechanism of endotoxin-induced diarrhea is not completely understood; however, it seems to involve both prostaglandins and nitric oxide. The administration of endotoxin leads to abundant accumulation of fluid inside the small intestines of animals, which is thought to be prostaglandin mediated.[4] Endotoxin also increases the enzyme activities of nitric oxide synthase in intestinal smooth muscle, which changes the propagation of jejunal contractions resulting in rapid intestinal transit.[5] The diarrhea observed during endotoxemia in cattle is not profuse but is generally described as low volume. In these cases, choosing to use an antimicrobial would likely not benefit the diarrhea or enteric disease present in the cows but would almost certainly be indicated from the standpoint of treating the primary disease condition.

Despite the limited number of enteric diseases in adult cattle that would benefit from antimicrobial therapy, surveys indicate that diarrhea is a relatively common reason for the use of antibiotics. In the 2007 National Animal Health Monitoring Survey (NAHMS) dairy study, mastitis was the most common reason for antimicrobial use on dairy farms followed by lameness, reproductive diseases (metritis), respiratory disease, and then diarrhea or other enteric disease. Results of the survey showed that about 2% of cattle on dairy farms from the survey population had been treated with an antimicrobial for diarrhea in the preceding 12-month period and 25% of farms said they routinely had cows that received antimicrobial drugs because of diarrhea.[6] Data from the NAHMS 2011 feedlot study indicated that 71% of feedlots reported diarrhea or other enteric disease in calves after arrival with 4.3% of calves showing evidence of diarrhea.[7] Further data from the study indicated that 54% of calves with diarrhea received treatment upon arrival. When the survey looked into what specific therapy was administered, 30% of calves received an injectable antimicrobial, while 51% of the cattle received an oral antibiotic. When reviewing the data of both the NAHMS dairy and feedlot studies, it becomes clear that enteric disease is not the primary reason for antimicrobial use in adult cattle. However, it is also apparent that diarrhea is one of the top 3 or 4 reasons cattle receive antimicrobials and that at least half of the cattle diagnosed with diarrhea receive either a parenteral and/or an oral antibiotic.

Most of the time dairy or beef cattle have diarrhea, it is not clear what the cause is, and therefore they are empirically treated with antibiotics. The assumption in many cases is that the animal has salmonellosis or some other bacterial enteritis. Although this is certainly true in some cases, it is very likely that most cases of diarrhea are because of simple indigestion caused by an abrupt diet change, moldy feed, spoiled feed, or perhaps a mild grain overload (rumen acidosis). However, simple indigestion is often difficult or impossible to diagnose definitively and therefore cattle are treated empirically with antimicrobials. If *Salmonella* are the main target of antimicrobial therapy in adult cattle with diarrhea, drug selection should ideally be based on the results of susceptibility testing using bacterial strains recovered from that particular dairy or feedlot. Broad-spectrum antimicrobials are usually used pending the availability of susceptibility test results. *Salmonella* show variable resistance patterns to ampicillin, amoxicillin, ceftiofur, florfenicol, neomycin, streptomycin, sulfonamides, tetracycline, and trimethoprim-sulfa and general resistance to penicillin, erythromycin, and tylosin.[8–10] The most recently published data indicated that *Salmonella* isolates from cattle were most commonly resistant to streptomycin, ampicillin, and sulfonamides, whereas resistance to ceftiofur was extremely low.[9] As *Salmonella* are facultative intracellular pathogens, selecting an antimicrobial with good tissue penetration and the ability to attain intracellular therapeutic drug concentrations within macrophages is desirable.

In summary, antimicrobials for the treatment of diarrhea in adult cattle are likely being overused at present in the cattle industry. Although diarrhea occurs fairly commonly, most causes are unlikely to respond to antimicrobials. Treatment should be primarily supportive care, including fluid therapy, anthelmintics if needed, and provision of good-quality pasture or other forages. Mortality rates in most cases of diarrhea in mature cattle are low, and the diarrhea generally resolves within a few days. Diseases such as paratuberculosis would have a higher mortality but would still not be likely to respond to antimicrobial therapy. However, when cattle have signs of systemic infection such as pyrexia or bloody diarrhea, it may be rational to begin antimicrobial therapy, particularly on farms that have a history of salmonellosis. When examining an adult ruminant with enteric disease, the practitioner should consider the age of the animal; the onset, severity, and duration of diarrhea (acute vs chronic); the number of cattle affected (is this an individual animal or a herd problem); clinical signs in the animal other than diarrhea (does the animal show systemic signs of disease); nutritional history (especially recent changes in the diet), and whether there has been an introduction of new animals (BVD). All these help to determine a list of possible causes for the diarrhea and may help reduce the use of antimicrobial drugs in cattle that are unlikely to benefit from therapy. Prudent use of antimicrobial drugs is recommended with an emphasis on establishing a herd diagnosis and conducting susceptibility testing for the specific *Salmonella* serotype or other bacterial pathogen present and choosing an appropriate antibiotic.

THE USE OF ANTIBIOTICS TO PREVENT CALF DIARRHEA

Calf health should be a priority on both beef and dairy farms. Despite this importance, the United States Department of Agriculture Dairy 2007 study shows a preweaned heifer calf mortality rate of 8.7% and reports that only 40% of farms can supply an adequate number of replacements from their own herd. Although mortality is slightly less in beef calves, 4% to 5% still die before weaning. In both beef and dairy calves, diarrhea represents the most common reason for loss due to death before weaning. Therefore, practitioners and producers spend a significant amount of time trying to prevent diarrhea and also making sure good treatment programs are in place when diarrhea does occur. The 3 main principles of diarrhea prevention in both beef and dairy cattle include (1) using a vaccine in late gestation cattle containing enterotoxigenic *Escherichia coli*, rotavirus, and coronavirus; (2) making sure a good colostrum program is in place ensuring adequate intake of immunoglobulins by the calf; and (3) decreasing the load of enteric pathogens in the environment through sanitation, hygiene, housing, and pasture management.

Historically, many producers (particularly in the dairy and veal industries) have used feeding of oral antibiotics to prevent diarrhea and hopefully decrease mortality in newborn calves. However, the practice of continually feeding antibiotics to calves is now prohibited in many countries, and the efficacy of feeding antibiotics to calves as a method of diarrhea prevention has not proven to be effective in recent studies. Almost 60 years ago, a thorough review was published on the efficacy of antibiotics for preventing diarrhea and improving weight gain in dairy calves.[11] The investigator concluded that the addition of chlortetracycline and oxytetracycline to milk replacer in the first 8 weeks of life decreased the incidence and severity of diarrhea. The minimum daily doses necessary for efficacy in this study were 0.15 to 0.20 mg/lb, which led to the routine inclusion of these antibiotics in milk replacers throughout the United States. Unfortunately, this study did not look at critical factors such as mortality rate in calves or incidence of diarrhea. The primary benefits of oral antibiotics were found to be higher weight gain and decreased severity and duration of diarrhea. As discussed in a previous review article, there were several studies done in the 1960s and the 1970s using various antibiotics (including ampicillin, chlortetracycline, furazolidone, neomycin, oxytetracycline, and streptomycin) to prevent diarrhea in calves.[12] Although the results of these studies varied, only 1 study documented a decrease in mortality rate from diarrhea due to prophylactic oral administration of chlortetracycline.[13] A few studies did find a decrease in the total number of days of diarrhea associated with antibiotics[12]; however, other studies (particularly with neomycin) found increased rates of diarrhea in antibiotic-treated calves.[14,15] Quite a few of these older studies found that oral administration of various antibiotics did not change the incidence of diarrhea in calves when compared with untreated controls.[16]

More recent studies have found that either oral antibiotics had no effect on decreasing calf diarrhea or in some cases diarrhea rates actually increased in calves fed antibiotics. For example, a study in California fed 1 group of Holstein heifers monensin in the starter ration, whereas another group was fed lasalocid and chlortetracycline (Aureomycin) for the first 12 weeks of life (in addition to nonmedicated milk replacer or whole milk). Antibiotic-treated calves had no difference in average daily gain, feed efficiency, or the proportion of calves treated for diarrhea.[17] In another study, Holstein heifers were fed milk replacer medicated with oxytetracycline and neomycin or an unmedicated milk replacer that contained a probiotic (Enteroguard—no longer commercially available). Once again, body weight gain, feed efficiency, and the incidence and severity of diarrhea were similar between groups.[18] In a third study, 358 dairy calves were divided into 4 groups: medicated milk replacer (neomycin and tetracycline for the first 14 days of life) plus the administration of trimethoprim-sulfamethoxazole, spectinomycin, penicillin, and bismuth pectin for the treatment of diarrhea (referred to as conventional therapy); medicated milk replacer for the first 14 days of life, bismuth pectin for diarrhea, and other antibiotics only in cases of fever or depressed attitude (targeted therapy); nonmedicated milk replacer with antimicrobial treatment of diarrhea (same treatments as the conventional therapy group above); and nonmedicated milk replacer with targeted therapy.[19] Calves fed a medicated milk replacer had 31% more days with diarrhea when compared with calves fed nonmedicated milk replacer.

In a 2007 survey, about 60% of dairy farms in the United States fed medicated milk replacers to preweaned heifer calves, most commonly a combination of oxytetracycline and neomycin.[6] However, a new federal regulation that began in 2010 restricts the feeding of medicated milk replacers to a period of 7 to 14 days. Thus continuous feeding of antibiotics in the milk from birth to weaning is no longer permitted, and this is meant to transition the use of oral antibiotics in calves from prophylactic to therapeutic. Medicated milk replacers should now be reserved for the treatment of bacterial enteritis (diarrhea) and bacterial pneumonia in dairy calves and not for prophylactic prevention. Since the late 1990s, the European Union has prohibited the sale of milk replacers and other animal feeds containing antibiotics. All the feed and milk replacers for dairy cattle must be sold as nonmedicated, and then antibiotics can be added only for therapeutic use (for example, in calves with diarrhea). Australia and New Zealand also have strict laws regarding the importation of any animal feed, and these products are generally nonmedicated as well. Overall, the conventional practice of adding antibiotics to milk or milk replacers for prophylactic use is being discouraged worldwide. Most modern studies fail to find any benefit of using antibiotics as a prevention for diarrhea, and their use in this manner should be discouraged.

THE RATIONALE FOR USING ANTIBIOTICS AS A TREATMENT OF CALF DIARRHEA

The use of antibiotics as a treatment in calves with diarrhea is a controversial topic with strong opinions on both sides. Several articles have been published indicating that antibiotics are contraindicated in calves with diarrhea or that they serve no beneficial purpose.[20,21] In contrast, other studies have indicated that antibiotics are effective in reducing mortality rate and speeding recovery in calves with diarrhea.[22,23] To begin the discussion, it is important to establish a reason to use antibiotics in calves with diarrhea. The 2 primary treatment goals of an antibiotic in calves with diarrhea would be (1) to prevent bacteremia and (2) to decrease the number of coliform bacteria in the small intestine.

Several studies have reported that a significant number of calves with diarrhea subsequently develop bacteremia. An initial study in the early 1960s reported that colostrum-deprived calves with diarrhea were frequently bacteremic (14/17 calves or 82%).[24] In contrast, none of the diarrheic calves in this study that had received colostrum were bacteremic (0.26 or 0%). A study conducted on a large calf-rearing facility in California examined 169 dairy calves with severe diarrhea[25]; 129 of the 169 calves (76%) had failure of passive transfer and 47 (28%) calves were bacteremic (predominantly *E coli*). Another study done in Prince Edward Island, Canada, looked at the prevalence of bacteremia in 252 calves with diarrhea[26]; 78 of the 252 (31%) calves in this study were bacteremic (predominantly *E coli*). As noted previously, the percentage of calves with bacteremia was significantly higher in the failure of passive transfer group (47/103 or 46%) than in adequate passive transfer group (21/116 or 18%). Taken together these studies indicate that it can be assumed that one-third of the calves with severe diarrhea are bacteremic and that the percentage is likely significantly higher in calves with failure of passive transfer. Although some have argued that antibiotic use in calves with diarrhea is inappropriate and leads to the emergence of resistant bacteria, a case can be made that the use of antibiotics to prevent and/or treat bacteremia in calves with diarrhea and systemic signs of disease is warranted. Withholding effective treatment (antibiotics) for a life-threatening disease (such as bacteremia in calves with diarrhea) should not be condoned on animal welfare grounds.[22]

Another potential reason for antibiotic therapy in calves with diarrhea is coliform overgrowth of the small intestine (**Fig. 1**). Research conducted in the 1920s documented increased numbers of *E coli* in the abomasum, duodenum, and jejunum of calves with diarrhea.[27,28] More recent studies have consistently found increased numbers of intestinal *E coli* in calves with naturally acquired diarrhea regardless of the age of the calf or the cause of the diarrhea.[29,30] Specifically, the numbers of *E coli* bacteria increase from 5- to 10,000-fold in the duodenum, jejunum, and ileum of calves with scours, even when rotavirus or coronavirus is identified as the cause of diarrhea.[22] This small intestinal overgrowth of the intestines with coliform bacteria can persist after the pathogen causing the diarrhea is gone.[30] The increased numbers of coliform bacteria in the small intestine of calves with diarrhea is associated with altered small intestinal function, morphologic damage, and increased susceptibility to bacteremia.[31] Therefore there is some logic to the use of antimicrobials in scouring calves to decrease the number of intestinal coliform bacteria. This use could potentially prevent the development of bacteremia, decrease calf mortality, and decrease damage to the small intestine, facilitating digestion and absorption and increasing growth rate.[22]

EFFICACY OF USING ANTIBIOTICS IN CALVES WITH DIARRHEA

An extensive review published in 2004 examined the question of whether or not antibiotics were effective in diarrheic calves.[22] This study reviewed articles published since 1950 and included studies with both orally and parenterally administered antibiotics in either naturally acquired or experimentally induced diarrhea. The investigator examined the effects of antibiotics on 4 critical measures of antimicrobial success in decreasing order of importance: (1) mortality rate, (2) growth rate in survivors, (3) severity of diarrhea in survivors, and (4) duration of diarrhea in survivors. The review looked at more than 20 different published studies involving a variety of antimicrobials,

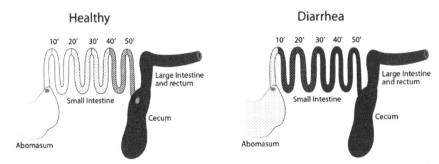

Fig. 1. Schematic of the distribution and concentration of *E coli* in the intestinal tract of a calf with undifferentiated diarrhea and a similarly aged calf without diarrhea. The figure indicates that the number of *E coli* in the large intestine of diarrheic and healthy calves is similar but that diarrheic calves have increased *E coli* numbers in their small intestine, particularly in the distal jejunum and ileum. (*Adapted from* Constable PD. Antimicrobial use in the treatment of calf diarrhea. J Vet Intern Med 2004;18:9.)

several of which would be illegal to use in the United States (ie, chloramphenicol, fura-zolidone, or marbofloxacin). The results indicated that specific antibiotics were effective in reducing mortality and increasing growth rate when administered to calves with diarrhea. Several studies provided evidence that even calves with simple diarrhea (without systemic signs of disease) seemed to recover faster with antibiotics as opposed to calves that did not receive antibiotics.

Some veterinarians feel that oral or parenteral administration of antibiotics to calves with diarrhea is contraindicated. The arguments most commonly used to support this approach include: (1) oral antibiotics alter intestinal flora and thereby induce diarrhea or exacerbate existing diarrhea, (2) antibiotics harm good intestinal bacteria more than bad bacteria, (3) antimicrobial use in calves with diarrhea is not effective, and (4) the use of antibiotics provides a selection pressure on the enteric bacterial population likely leading to increased antimicrobial resistance.[22] There is solid evidence to indicate that the use of antimicrobial drugs can decrease mortality in calves and there is no evidence to support the argument that antimicrobials harm good bacteria more than the bad. However, the emergence of resistant bacteria is certainly serious and is something the veterinarian must take into account before treating calves with diarrhea.

WHICH ANTIBIOTICS SHOULD BE USED IN CALVES WITH DIARRHEA

Table 1 contains a list of antimicrobials currently approved for the treatment or prevention of diarrhea in the United States. At present, oxytetracycline administered parenterally and chlortetracycline, neomycin, oxytetracycline, sulfamethazine, and tetracycline administered orally are the only antimicrobials labeled in the United States for the treatment of calf diarrhea. Of these, none have been shown to be consistently efficacious in peer-reviewed studies. As discussed above, when treating calves with diarrhea the 2 primary goals of therapy are to (1) decrease the number of E coli bacteria in the small intestine and (2) treat potential E coli bacteremia. With these goals in mind, the target of antimicrobial therapy in calves with diarrhea should be coliform bacteria both in the blood and in the small intestine.

As none of the approved drugs for treating diarrhea in the United States are likely to be effective, extralabel use is likely justified. Some efficacy has been described for oral amoxicillin in the treatment of calves with experimentally induced diarrhea,[16,32] but was not effective in the treatment of naturally acquired diarrhea in beef calves.[33] Amoxicillin trihydrate (10 mg/kg administered orally every 12 h) or amoxicillin trihydrate-clavulanate (12.5 mg combined drug/kg administered orally every 12 h) for at least 3 days is one antimicrobial approach that likely has some efficacy for calves with diarrhea. Amoxicillin is partially absorbed from the calf small intestine with absorption being similar in both milk-fed and fasted calves.[34] High amoxicillin concentrations are found in bile and intestinal contents after oral administration, with lower concentrations in serum.[32] Oral ampicillin could also be used, and its efficacy in one study was shown to be equivalent to that of amoxicillin.[35] Although very popular in the United States, oral sulfonamides cannot be recommended for treating calves with diarrhea because of the lack of efficacy studies. Most antimicrobial susceptibility studies done in the past 30 years indicate that sulfamethazine (and other sulfonamide drugs) would have poor sensitivity against coliform bacteria in the blood or small intestine.

The most logical antimicrobial for parenteral treatment of calf diarrhea in the United States is ceftiofur (2.2 mg/kg given intramuscularly [IM] every 12 h) for at least 3 days. Ceftiofur is a broad-spectrum antibiotic that is resistant to β-lactamase. The labeled

Table 1
Antibiotics approved in the United States for control and/or treatment of calf diarrhea

Antibiotic	Trade Name	Manufacturer	Label Claim	Dose
Chlortetracycline	Aureomycin soluble powder concentrate	Zoetis	Control and treatment of scours caused by E coli or Salmonella spp	22 mg/kg of body weight for 3–5 d orally
Chlortetracycline	Aureomycin 90 Granular or Aureomycin 90 Meal or CLTC 100 MR	Zoetis or Phibro	Treatment of scours caused by E coli	22 mg/kg of body weight mixed or top dressed on feed daily for up to 5 d
Chlortetracycline	ChlorMax 50	Zoetis	Treatment of scours caused by E coli	22 mg/kg of body weight in milk replacer or starter feeds for up to 5 d
Neomycin	Neomed 325 soluble powder	Bimeda	Control and treatment of scours caused by E coli	22 mg/kg of body weight mixed in drinking water, maximum of 14 d
Neomycin	Neomycin oral solution	AgriLabs	Control and treatment of scours caused by E coli	22 mg/kg of body weight given orally divided into at least 2 doses per day, maximum of 14 d
Neomycin-Oxytetracycline	Neo-Terramycin 50/50 or Neo-Terramycin 100/100	Phibro	Treatment of E coli diarrhea	22 mg/kg of body weight fed continuously for a maximum of 14 d
Neomycin-Oxytetracycline	NT concentrate	Land O'Lakes	Treatment and control of E coli diarrhea	Mix in milk replacer to deliver 22 mg/kg of body weight fed continuously for a maximum of 14 d
Oxytetracycline	300 Pro LA	Norbrook	Treatment of E coli diarrhea	6.6–11 mg/kg of body weight daily IM or SC for up to 4 d
Oxytetracycline	Agrimycin 200 or Bio-Mycin 200 or Duramycin 72–200	AgriLabs, Boehringer Ingelheim, or Durvet	Treatment of E coli diarrhea	6.6–11 mg/kg of body weight daily IM or SC for up to 4 d

Antimicrobial	Trade Name	Manufacturer	Indication	Dosage
Oxytetracycline	Calf scours bolus	Durvet	Control and treatment of scours caused by E coli or Salmonella typhimurium	250 mg/45.4 kg of body weight orally every 12 h for up to 4 d (control) or 500 mg every 12 h (treatment)
Oxytetracycline	Terramycin Scours Tablet or Oxy 500 Calf Bolus	Zoetis or Boehringer Ingelheim	Control and treatment of scours caused by E coli or Salmonella typhimurium	5.5 mg/kg of body weight orally every 12 h for up to 4 d (control) or 5 mg/lb every 12 h (treatment)
Oxytetracycline	Terramycin 50, 100, or 200; Terramycin 200 Granular, or Terramycin 100 MR	Phibro	Treatment of E coli diarrhea	22 mg/kg of body weight fed continuously for 7–14 d
Sulfamethazine	SMZ-Med 454 or Sulmet Powder	Bimeda or Boehringer Ingelheim	Treatment of E coli diarrhea	238 mg/kg of body weight on day 1 followed by 119 mg/kg on days 2, 3, and 4, mixed in water
Sulfamethazine	Sulmet Oblets	Boehringer Ingelheim	Treatment of E coli diarrhea	220 mg/kg of body weight on day 1 (given orally) followed by 110 mg/kg on days 2, 3 and 4
Sulfamethazine	Sustain III Boluses	Bimeda, or Durvet, or VetOne	Treatment of E coli scours	352 mg/kg of body weight given orally, given once every 3 d for a maximum of 2 treatments
Tetracycline	Duramycin-10	Durvet	Control scours caused by E coli	Dissolve in drinking water to provide daily dose of 22 mg/kg of body weight for up to 3–5 d
Tetracycline	Tet-Sol 324, Tetramed 324 HCA, Tetra Bac 324, or PolyOtic soluble powder	Zoetis, Bimeda, AgriLabs, or Boehringer Ingelheim	Control and treatment of E coli diarrhea	Dissolve in drinking water to provide daily dose of 22 mg/kg of body weight for up to 3–5 d

The list of trade names is not necessarily complete.
Abbreviations: IM, intramuscularly; SC, subcutaneously.

dose maintains plasma concentrations of ceftiofur above the minimum concentration required to inhibit the growth of 90% of E coli (MIC_{90}) in young calves (0.25 µg/mL). Furthermore, 30% of the active metabolite (desfuroylceftiofur) is excreted into the intestinal tract of cattle providing activity in both the blood and the small intestine. Parenteral ampicillin (10 mg/kg IM every 12 h) is another antibiotic that would be likely to have efficacy in calves with diarrhea. In Europe, parenteral enrofloxacin is labeled for the treatment of calf diarrhea, and several studies have documented efficacy with using fluoroquinolone antibiotics in calves with diarrhea.[36–38] However, it must be emphasized that the extralabel use of fluoroquinolone antibiotics in the United States is illegal and obviously not recommended. Historically, gentamicin was also considered an appropriate treatment for use in calves with diarrhea. However, parenteral administration of aminoglycosides cannot be recommended in calves with diarrhea because of the lack of published efficacy studies, prolonged slaughter withdrawal times (18 months), potential for nephrotoxicity in dehydrated calves, and availability of other drugs likely to be equally successful (ceftiofur, amoxicillin, and ampicillin).

The issue of whether or not to use antibiotics in a calf with simple diarrhea (without systemic signs of disease) is a little more controversial. Although there have been studies to show that these calves gain more weight and recover faster than calves not given antibiotics,[22] there are other studies that indicate no benefit to using antibiotics in these cases.[19,20] The clinician must weigh any potential benefit of antimicrobial therapy against the possibility of increasing the population of resistant bacteria on the farm. A fairly recent study demonstrated that individual treatment of sick calves with antibiotics increased the level of resistance to E coli isolates; however, the change in antimicrobial susceptibility was only transient.[39]

ANTIMICROBIAL SUSCEPTIBILITY TESTING

The next logical question is whether or not antimicrobial susceptibility testing should play a role in determining which drug is used to treat calves with diarrhea. Historically, culture and susceptibility results from fecal culture have been routinely used to guide treatment decisions; however, it is not clear whether or not this has any clinical relevance. Research validating susceptibility testing as being predictive of treatment outcome for calves with diarrhea is currently not available. Part of the problem is that our target is coliform bacteria in the blood and small intestine, which are likely different from fecal bacterial flora. Older studies have demonstrated that the predominant strain of E coli in the manure of calves with diarrhea usually changes several times during the course of disease.[24,40] These studies also show that about 50% of calves have different E coli strains isolated from the upper and lower parts of small intestine.[24] So it is logical to conclude that fecal coliform isolates are not representative of what is happening in the intestine.

Another potential problem with using susceptibility testing to guide antimicrobial selection in cases of diarrhea is that most of the bacterial cultures submitted usually come from dead animals, which represent treatment failures and may have already received antibiotics. Preferential growth of resistant bacterial strains can start within a few hours after antibiotic administration, and therefore culture results from dead calves may not be representative of the actual clinical problem.[41] To the author's knowledge, the only study that has tried to assess the predictive ability of fecal antimicrobial susceptibility testing found that it was an inaccurate predictor of clinical outcome.[42] In a large group of experiments evaluating the efficacy of amoxicillin for treating calf diarrhea, 205 calves were divided into groups that either received amoxicillin or did not. Diarrhea was experimentally induced using enterotoxigenic E coli and rectal swab culture, and susceptibility testing was done. Most calves (80%) developed diarrhea after challenge; however, in only about 25% of cases did calves shed the actual challenge strain of *E coli*. Recovery or treatment success in these studies was defined as normal feces within 4 days after the start of treatment, while treatment failure was defined as death or scouring for more than 4 days. Among calves in which the *E coli* cultured from rectal swabs were susceptible to amoxicillin, 10% died and 62% recovered with 3.3 as the mean number of days scouring. Outcomes were not different in calves that had amoxicillin-resistant strains of *E coli* cultured from rectal swabs with 12% death loss, 60% recovery rates, and 3.6 scouring days. In calves given a placebo instead of amoxicillin, mortality was significantly increased (20%), recovery rates were decreased (34%), and the number of scouring days was longer (5.1). The investigators concluded that amoxicillin had a significant effect on disease by decreasing mortality and number of scouring days; however, treatment success could not be predicted by whether the *E coli* cultured from rectal swabs was susceptible or resistant to the antimicrobial being used.

Two studies have concluded that there was a good correlation between in vitro antimicrobial susceptibility of fecal *E coli* isolates and clinical response to treatment; however, neither study had data to statistically analyze this association.[43,44] In contrast, 2 other studies reported no correlation between in vitro susceptibility results for coliform isolates and response to antimicrobial treatment.[45,46] However, these studies did not differentiate enterotoxigenic and nonenterotoxigenic strains of *E coli* and also failed to do any statistical analysis of the data. There is a significant need for antimicrobial susceptibility data from *E coli* and *Salmonella* isolates collected from the small intestine of untreated calves with diarrhea. Minimum inhibitory concentrations (MIC) could then be compared with free antimicrobial concentrations that are actually achievable in the intestinal tract of calves to determine the best drug to use along with the optimal dosing interval. However, it should be emphasized that antimicrobial concentrations can be altered by multiple variables, such as intestinal pH, which may be quite different between healthy calves and those with diarrhea. Therefore even after establishing MIC values and setting appropriate breakpoints, these need to be validated through clinical trials examining the use of specific antimicrobial drugs in calves with diarrhea as compared to the pathogen isolated and disease outcome. Until then the use of fecal culture and susceptibility testing to guide antimicrobial selection for treating calf diarrhea is probably of little value. Drug selection is based on knowledge of the likely pathogen (*E coli* in the blood and small intestine), pharmacokinetics of the drug (can it achieve therapeutic concentrations at the site of infection), and evaluation of the response to treatment (does the animal get better). On farms in which *Salmonella* or *E coli* septicemia is a problem, looking at susceptibility results from blood cultures is likely much more appropriate than fecal culture.

Certainly the overuse of antibiotics is a concern, and the overall philosophy in veterinary medicine is to use antibiotics conservatively to preserve the efficacy of these drugs in both animals and humans. Based on the need to minimize the use of antibiotics and because of the lack of any demonstrated recent efficacy, the feeding of antimicrobials to calves as a method of diarrhea prevention is not recommended. However, calves with diarrhea and systemic signs of illness should receive antibiotics targeted toward coliform bacteria in the blood (because of likelihood of bacteremia) and the small intestine (because of bacterial overgrowth). A clinical sepsis scoring system to predict bacteremia based on physical examination does not seem to be sufficiently accurate to guide antimicrobial decision making, and therefore the clinician should assume that calves are bacteremic when they exhibit inappetence, dehydration, lethargy, or fever. In calves with diarrhea and no systemic signs of illness (normal appetite for milk, no fever), evidence suggests that the clinician continue to monitor the health of the calf and not administer antibiotics unless the calf's condition deteriorates.

REFERENCES

1. Shahriar FM, Clark EG, Janzen E, et al. Coinfection with bovine viral diarrhea virus and *Mycoplasma bovis* in feedlot cattle with chronic pneumonia. Can Vet J 2002; 43:863–8.
2. Daly RF, Neiger RD. Outbreak of *Salmonella enterica* serotype newport in a beef cow-calf herd associated with exposure to bovine viral diarrhea virus. J Am Vet Med Assoc 2008;233:618–23.
3. Smith GW. Supportive therapy of the toxic cow. Vet Clin North Am Food Anim Pract 2005;21:595–614.
4. Liang YC, Liu HJ, Chen SH, et al. Effect of lipopolysaccharide on diarrhea and gastrointestinal transit in mice: roles of nitric oxide and prostaglandin E_2. World J Gastroenterol 2005;11:357–61.
5. Cullen JJ, Mercer D, Hinkhouse M, et al. Effects of endotoxin on regulation of intestinal smooth muscle nitric oxide synthase and intestinal transit. Surgery 1999; 125:339–44.
6. United States Department of Agriculture Animal Plant Health Inspection Service (USDA APHIS). Antibiotic use on US dairy operations, 2002 and 2007. 2008. Available at: http://www.aphis.usda.gov/animal_health/nahms/dairy/downloads/dairy07/Dairy07_is_AntibioticUse.pdf. Accessed September 9, 2014.
7. United States Department of Agriculture Animal Plant Health Inspection Service (USDA APHIS). Feedlot 2011 Part IV: health and health management on U.S. feedlots with a capacity of 1,000 or more head. 2013. Available at: http://www.aphis.usda.gov/animal_health/nahms/feedlot/downloads/feedlot2011/Feed11_dr_PartIV.pdf. Accessed September 9, 2014.
8. Mohler VL, Izzo MM, House JK. *Salmonella* in calves. Vet Clin North Am Food Anim Pract 2009;25:37–54.
9. Izzo MM, Mohler VL, House JK. Antimicrobial susceptibility of *Salmonella* isolates recovered from calves with diarrhea in Australia. Aust Vet J 2011;89:402–8.
10. Ray KA, Warnick LD, Mithcell RM, et al. Prevalence of antimicrobial resistance among *Salmonella* on midwest and northeast USA dairy farms. Prev Vet Med 2007;79:204–23.
11. Lassiter CA. Antibiotics as growth stimulants for dairy cattle: a review. J Dairy Sci 1955;38:1102–8.
12. Constable PD. Use of antibiotics to prevent calf diarrhea and septicemia. Bovine Pract 2003;37:137–42.
13. Dalton RG, Fisher EW, McIntyre WI. Antibiotics and calf diarrhea. Vet Rec 1960; 72:1186–99.
14. Rollin RE, Mero KN, Kozisek PB, et al. Diarrhea and malabsorption in calves associated with therapeutic doses of antibiotics: absorptive and clinical changes. Am J Vet Res 1986;47:987–91.
15. Shull JJ, Frederick HM. Adverse effect of oral antibacterial prophylaxis and therapy on incidence of neonatal calf diarrhea. Vet Med Small Anim Clin 1978;73:924–30.
16. Bywater J. Evaluation of an oral glucose-glycine-electrolyte formulation and amoxicillin for the treatment of diarrhea in calves. Am J Vet Res 1977;38:1983–7.

17. Higginbotham GE, Pereira LN, Chebel RC, et al. A field trial comparing the effects of supplementation with Aureomycin plus lasalocid or monensin on the health and production performance of dairy calves. Prof Anim Sci 2010;26:520–6.

18. Donovan DC, Franklin ST, Chase CC, et al. Growth and health of Holstein calves fed milk replacers supplemented with antibiotics or Enteroguard. J Dairy Sci 2002;85:947–50.

19. Berge AC, Moore DA, Besser TE, et al. Targeting therapy to minimize antimicrobial use in preweaned calves: effects on health, growth, and treatment costs. J Dairy Sci 2009;92:4707–14.

20. de Verdier K, Ohagen P, Alenius S, et al. No effect of a homeopathic preparation on neonatal calf diarrhea in a randomized double-blind, placebo-controlled clinical trial. Acta Vet Scand 2003;44:97–101.

21. Grove-White DH. A rational approach to treatment of calf diarrhea. Ir Vet J 2004; 57:722–8.

22. Constable PD. Antimicrobial use in the treatment of calf diarrhea. J Vet Intern Med 2004;18:8–17.

23. Constable PD. Treatment of calf diarrhea: antimicrobial and ancillary treatments. Vet Clin North Am Food Anim Pract 2009;25:101–20.

24. Smith HW. Observations on the etiology of neonatal diarrhea (scours) in calves. J Pathol Bacteriol 1962;84:147–68.

25. Fecteau G, Van Metre DC, Pare J, et al. Bacteriological culture of blood from critically ill neonatal calves. Can Vet J 1997;38:95–100.

26. Loftstedt J, Dohoo IR, Duizer G. Model to predict septicemia in diarrheic calves. J Vet Intern Med 1999;13:81–8.

27. Carpenter CM, Woods G. The distribution of the colon-aerogenes group of bacteria in the alimentary tract of calves. Cornell Vet 1924;14:218–25.

28. Smith T, Orcutt ML. The bacteriology of the intestinal tract of young calves with special reference to early diarrhea. J Exp Med 1925;41:89–106.

29. Issacson RE, Moon HW, Schneider RA. Distribution and virulence of *Escherichia coli* in the small intestine of calves with and without diarrhea. Am J Vet Res 1978; 39:1750–5.

30. Youanes YD, Herdt TH. Changes in small intestinal morphology and flora associated with decreased energy digestibility in calves with naturally occurring diarrhea. Am J Vet Res 1987;48:719–25.

31. Reisinger RC. Pathogenesis and prevention of infectious diarrhea (scours) of newborn calves. J Am Vet Med Assoc 1965;147:1377–86.

32. Palmer GH, Bywater RJ, Francis ME. Amoxycillin: distribution and clinical efficacy in calves. Vet Rec 1977;100:487–91.

33. Radostits OM, Rhodes CS, Mitchell ME, et al. A clinical evaluation of antimicrobial agents and temporary starvation in the treatment of acute undifferentiated diarrhea in newborn calves. Can Vet J 1975;16:219–27.

34. Ziv G, Nouws JF, Groothuis DG, et al. Oral absorption and bioavailability of ampicillin derivatives in calves. Am J Vet Res 1977;38:1007–13.

35. Keefe TJ. Clinical efficacy of amoxicillin in calves with colibacillosis. Vet Med Small Anim Clin 1977;72(Suppl):783–6.

36. Thomas E, Gruet P, Davot JL, et al. Field evaluation of efficacy of marbofloxacin bolus in the treatment of naturally occurring diarrhea in the new born calf. In: Abstracts of the 20th World Buiatrics Congress. Sydney, July 6–10, 1998. p. 337–9.

37. White DG, Johnson CK, Cracknell V. Comparison of danofloxacin with baquiloprim/sulphadimidine for the treatment of experimentally induced *Escherichia coli* diarrhea in calves. Vet Rec 1998;143:273–6.

38. Sunderland SJ, Sarasola P, Rowan TG, et al. Efficacy of danofloxacin 18% inject-able solution in the treatment of *Escherichia coli* diarrhoea in young calves in Europe. Res Vet Sci 2003;74:171–8.

39. Berge AC, Moore DA, Sischo WM, et al. Field trial evaluating the influence of prophylactic and therapeutic antimicrobial administration on antimicrobial resis-tance of fecal *Escherichia coli* in dairy calves. Appl Environ Microbiol 2006;72: 3872–8.

40. Smith HW, Crabb WE. The typing of *E. coli* by bacteriophage, its application to the study of *E. coli* populations of the intestinal tract of healthy calves and of calves suffering from white scours. J Gen Microbiol 1956;15:556–74.

41. Mylrea PJ. Passage of antibiotics through the digestive tract of normal and scour-ing calves and their effect upon the bacterial flora. Res Vet Sci 1968;9:5–13.

42. Bywater RJ, Palmer GH, Wanstall SA. Discrepancy between antibiotic (amoxy-cillin) resistance in vitro and efficacy in calf diarrhea. Vet Rec 1978;102:150–1.

43. Smith HW. Further observations on the effect of chemotherapy on the presence of drug-resistant *Bacterium coli* in the intestinal tract of calves. Vet Rec 1958;70: 575–80.

44. Smith HW, Crabb WE. The sensitivity to chemotherapeutic agents of a further series of strains of *Bacterium coli* from cases of white scours: the relationship between sensitivity tests and response to treatment. Vet Rec 1956;68:274–7.

45. Boyd JW, Baker JR, Leyland A, et al. Neonatal diarrhea in calves. Vet Rec 1974; 95:310–3.

46. Glantz PJ, Kradel DC, Seward SA. *Escherichia coli* and *Salmonella newport* in calves: efficacy of prophylactic and therapeutic treatment. Vet Med Small Anim Clin 1974;69:77–82.

Infectious Bovine Keratoconjunctivitis (Pinkeye)

John A. Angelos, MS, DVM, PhD

KEYWORDS

- Pinkeye • Infectious bovine keratoconjunctivitis • *Moraxella bovis*
- *Moraxella bovoculi* • Treatment • Prevention

KEY POINTS

- Effective treatment of pinkeye requires accurate diagnosis.
- Antibiotic treatment can shorten the healing time.
- Multiple routes of antibiotic delivery can be effective.
- Efforts to develop herd preventive strategies must involve consideration of risk factors.

Video of classic signs of infectious bovine keratoconjunctivitis and healing following treatment accompanies this article at http://www.vetfood.theclinics.com/

INTRODUCTION

Infectious bovine keratoconjunctivitis (IBK or "pinkeye") is the most common eye disease of cattle and can affect all breeds; however, a greater incidence of disease has been reported in lighter-colored breeds, such as Hereford or Hereford-crossbred cattle.[1–4] The etiologic agent of IBK is considered to be the gram-negative rod-shaped organism named *Moraxella bovis*. The pathogenicity of *Mor bovis* requires the expression of pilin for attachment to the ocular surface[5,6] and a cytotoxin[7] that damages corneal epithelial cells both in vitro[8] and in vivo.[9,10] Although a 2007 report of *Moraxella bovoculi*[11] isolated from eyes of calves affected with IBK has led to increased diagnoses of *Mor bovoculi* from ocular swabs of cattle with clinical IBK, experimental challenge studies have failed to demonstrate a role for *Mor bovoculi* in causing corneal ulcers associated with IBK.[12] Nevertheless, the identification of both a cytotoxin in *Mor bovoculi*[13] and more recently a putative pilin gene[14] warrant further investigations into the role that *Mor bovoculi* may play in IBK. It is possible that *Mor bovoculi* may play a role similar to other pathogens such as *Mycoplasma* spp and infectious bovine rhinotracheitis (IBR; bovine herpesvirus) that induce ocular pathologic abnormality and may assist in *Mor bovis*–associated ocular colonization or spread.[15–18] In this

Department of Medicine and Epidemiology, University of California, 2108 Tupper Hall, Davis, CA 95616, USA
E-mail address: jaangelos@ucdavis.edu

Vet Clin Food Anim 31 (2015) 61–79
http://dx.doi.org/10.1016/j.cvfa.2014.11.006
0749-0720/15/$ – see front matter © 2015 Elsevier Inc. All rights reserved.
vetfood.theclinics.com

article, both *Mor bovis* and *Mor bovoculi* are included in the discussion because both organisms are commonly isolated from cattle with IBK and treatment is often sought for one or both of these organisms. Nevertheless, studies published to date have not proven a direct causal role for *Mor bovoculi* in IBK.[12]

Colonization of the eyes of cattle by *Mor bovis*[19,20] and *Mor bovoculi* (John A. Angelos, MS, DVM, PhD, personal observation, 2008) can occur in the absence of clinical disease and both organisms can be cultured from the eyes of healthy cattle. Exactly what other intrinsic factors are that might play a role in stimulating otherwise commensal *Moraxella* spp to cause disease are not well understood; however, during efforts to control an outbreak of IBK, it is important to consider the role that extrinsic risk factors can play in IBK development. Such factors include exposure to ultraviolet radiation,[19,21,22] flies,[23–26] *Mycoplasma* spp infection,[17,18] IBR virus infection,[15,16] and foreign bodies (dust, plant awns). The typical pattern of fluorescein dye staining of a cornea damaged by a plant awn such as a foxtail (**Fig. 1**) embedded in the soft tissues surrounding the globe is that of uniform uptake to the corneal-scleral junction (**Fig. 2**).

Published reports of *Mycoplasma* spp in ocular lesions identified clinically as IBK with no evidence of *Mor bovis*[27–29] help to underscore why it is important to submit appropriate diagnostic specimens on appropriate test media to clinical microbiology laboratories when trying to establish a cause for ocular lesions presumed to be IBK. It is also a good idea to consult with your clinical microbiology laboratory in advance of sample collection to determine the best sample to collect and media to use for sample transport. This relatively small investment in time can pay large dividends later by saving veterinarians and their clients both time and money. Opinions on the use and efficacy of autogenous vaccines to prevent IBK vary widely; however, if a client has expressed interest in the development of an autogenous vaccine, it would be important to request the clinical microbiology laboratory to preserve isolates for such use during initial sample submission.

PATIENT EVALUATION OVERVIEW

A close-up examination of the bovine eye usually requires the animal to be restrained in a chute, often with a halter to properly position the animal's head. Thorough examination of the eye to investigate for the presence of foreign bodies will require rotation of the head and close animal contact, especially in instances where a foreign body is suspected based on the pattern of fluorescein staining when no plant fibers are immediately visible. During such examinations and especially with cattle exhibiting severe epiphora, ocular secretions harboring *Moraxella* spp can easily soak into the clothing

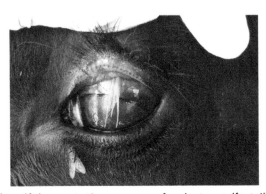

Fig. 1. Left eye of a calf demonstrating presence of a plant awn (foxtail).

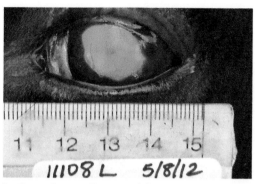

Fig. 2. Same eye as in **Fig. 1** after application of fluorescein dye. Note the staining pattern where the area of fluorescein dye uptake is continuous with the corneal-scleral junction; this pattern is characteristic of a foreign body–associated corneal ulcer.

of animal handlers and veterinarians performing such examinations. For these reasons, it is recommended to wear gloves and, if possible, an impervious apron or other nonabsorbing type of clothing that can be disinfected with dilute bleach or chlorhexidine between animals. In addition to hands and clothing, halters should be disinfected between animals as well as any equipment used to examine the eye, such as forceps used for removal of foreign bodies.

Classic signs of IBK include corneal ulceration and opacity (edema), photophobia, blepharospasm, lacrimation, and epiphora (**Fig. 3**, Video 1). Early lesions can be extremely small and easily missed (**Fig. 4**), and clear evidence of corneal edema may be difficult to appreciate from a distance. In these animals, the presence of epiphora and slight photophobia and blepharospasm can provide early clues to the presence of disease. As IBK progresses, other clinical signs, including increased corneal opacity and worsening blepharospasm, photophobia, and epiphora, will develop (**Figs. 5–8**). Most corneal ulcerations associated with IBK will heal with varying degrees of corneal scarring that can impair vision (**Fig. 9**). The ocular pain associated with IBK along with reduced vision and subsequent reduced feed intake most likely account for reduced weight gains in cattle with IBK.[2,30–32] In the most severe cases, corneal rupture can occur, resulting in permanent blindness (**Fig. 10**). Globe healing can occur following ocular rupture (**Fig. 11**); calves with such protruberant-appearing globes during severe inflammation are often referred to by producers as "popeyes."

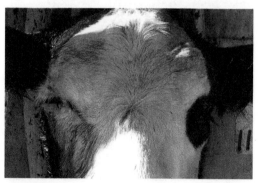

Fig. 3. Calf with IBK; the right eye has been stained with fluorescein dye. Note the presence of lacrimation, epiphora, and ocular pain in the right eye.

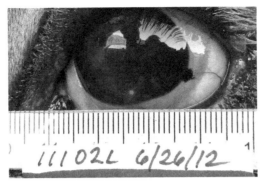

Fig. 4. Early IBK lesion in a calf. Note the approximately 1-mm-diameter focal area of fluorescein dye uptake at the 6 o'clock position. Early IBK lesions can be difficult to identify, and use of other clinical signs such as excessive lacrimation, epiphora, and/or blepharospasm/photophobia may be helpful to identify such cases.

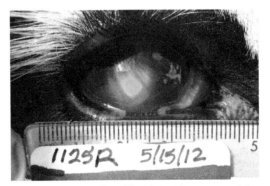

Fig. 5. Close-up view of the right eye of a calf with IBK. Two areas of fluorescein staining are present along with corneal edema, and whitish-yellow appearance to stromal layers that indicate infiltration of white blood cells.

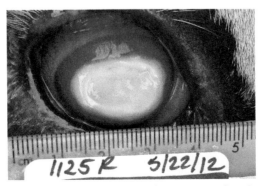

Fig. 6. Same eye as in **Fig. 5**, 1 week later. Note the presence of ocular inflammation and ingrowth of blood vessels that indicates that active healing is taking place. The calf in this photo was treated with 40 mg/kg florfenicol SC on the day that this photo was taken.

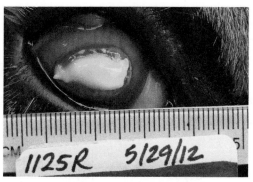

Fig. 7. Same eye as in **Fig. 6**, 1 week later. Note that healing is ongoing as evidenced by the continued ingrowth of blood vessels toward the center of the corneal injury.

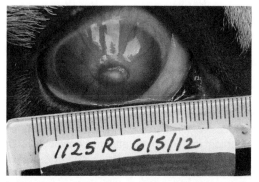

Fig. 8. Same eye as in **Fig. 7**, 1 week later. Overall, the inflammation remains most active at the center of the lesion and is resolving closer to the limbus.

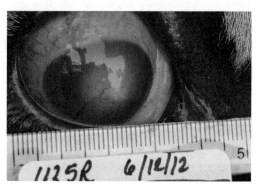

Fig. 9. Same eye as in **Fig. 8**, 1 week later. Blood vessels appear to have bridged the site of the original ulcer. At this time, the eye, although still cloudy, was much quieter and the calf seemed comfortable.

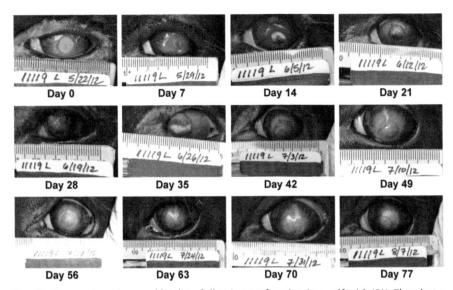

Fig. 10. Progression of corneal healing following perforation in a calf with IBK. The photographs depict a 77-day time frame. The calf was treated with florfenicol (40 mg/kg SC) on day 0 when the ulcer was first identified. Although the globe healed, the calf was permanently blind in the affected eye.

PHARMACOLOGIC TREATMENT OPTIONS

IBK research reported over the past approximately 60 years has led to conclusions that a variety of antibiotics administered via intramuscular (IM), subcutaneous (SC), subconjunctival, and topical routes can be effective against IBK. Unfortunately, there

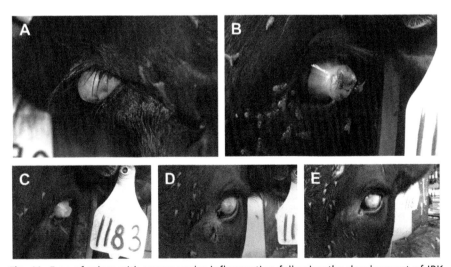

Fig. 11. Eyes of calves with severe ocular inflammation following the development of IBK and likely rupture of the globe. (A, B) Two different calves with lesions described by producers as "popeyes." (C–E) Calf depicted in (B) during the subsequent 3 weeks at each weekly interval. This calf received florfenicol (40 mg/kg SC) one time on the day that the photo in (B) was taken.

has been a lack of randomization and adequate controls in many of these published studies; this finding underscores the need for better study designs for future studies that evaluate treatments for IBK.[33] At the present time in the United States, only 2 parenterally administered antibiotics carry label claims to treat IBK because of *Mor bovis*: oxytetracycline and tulathromycin. In the event that approved treatments prove ineffective against IBK in some herds, however, legal routes to the use of alternate antibiotics exist through the Animal Medicinal Drug Use Clarification Act (AMDUCA) and its implementing regulations published at Title 21, Code of Federal Regulations, Part 530 (21 CFR 530).[34,35] Many of the drugs and drug formulations that have been evaluated for efficacy against IBK are not currently available in the United States and the following discussion on treatment focuses on those drugs, formulations, and preparations that would be most accessible to US practitioners.

Moraxella bovis and *Mor bovoculi* are generally considered to be susceptible to a variety of different antibiotics. In the case of *Mor bovis*, the organism is known to survive in or on ocular surfaces, a fact that rationalizes the widely practiced method of sampling ocular fluids for bacterial culture (ie, the swabbing of conjunctival fluid/ocular surfaces). To help reduce nonspecific contamination and improve chances of isolating *Moraxella* spp when collecting ocular fluid samples, it is recommended to swab the edges of corneal ulcers rather than the subconjunctival fornix (K. Clothier, DVM, PhD, California Animal Health and Food Safety Laboratory; personal communication, 2012). In experimental and natural IBK infections, *Mor bovis* is also found to exist within the corneal stroma.[10,36] To reach these surfaces adequately to assist in clearing an infection, an antibiotic would have to be delivered directly locally in the eye and/or by methods that ensure delivery of antibiotic via ocular fluid secretions.

Table 1 (for *Mor bovis*[37]) and **Table 2** (for *Mor bovoculi*[38]) list antibiotic concentrations tested and breakpoints used in determining the minimum inhibitory concentrations (MIC) of selected antibiotics necessary to inhibit 90% of isolates (MIC$_{90}$) by

Table 1
Concentrations and breakpoints used for antibiotics tested against 88 isolates of *Moraxella bovis* from Argentina

Antimicrobial Agent	Concentration Range Tested (µg/mL)	MIC Breakpoint (µg/mL)		
		Sensitive	Intermediate	Resistant
Ampicillin	0.25–32	≤0.25	8	≥16
Ceftiofur	0.06–8	≤2	4	≥8
Enrofloxacin	0.03–4	≤0.5	1	≥2
Erythromycin	0.12–16	≤0.5	1	≥8
Florfenicol	0.12–16	≤2	4	≥8
Gentamicin	0.5–32	≤4	8	≥16
Lincomycin	0.25–32	≤0.5	1	≥4
Oxytetracycline	0.5–32	≤4	8	≥16
Spectinomycin	1–128	≤32	64	≥128
Tilmicosin	0.25–32	≤8	16	≥32
Trimethoprim/Sulfamethoxazole	0.25/4.75–15/304	≤2/38		≥4/76
Tylosin	0.5–64	a	a	a

[a] No defined breakpoints.

Data from Zielinski G, Piscitelli H, Perez-Monti H, et al. Antibiotic sensitivity of an Argentine strain collection of Moraxella bovis. Vet Ther 2000;1:199–204.

Table 2
Concentrations and breakpoints used for antibiotics tested against 57 isolates of *Moraxella bovoculi* from cattle with infectious bovine keratoconjunctivitis in California from 2002 through 2007

Antimicrobial Agent	Concentration Range Tested (µg/mL)	MIC Breakpoint (µg/mL)		
		Sensitive	Intermediate	Resistant
Ampicillin	0.25–16	≤8	16	≥32
Ceftiofur[a]	0.25–8	≤2	4	≥8
Chlortetracycline	0.5–8	≤2	4	≥8
Clindamycin	0.25–16	≤0.5	1–2	≥4
Danofloxacin[a]	0.12–1	≤0.25	b	b
Enrofloxacin[a]	0.12–2	≤0.25	0.5–1	≥2
Florfenicol[a]	0.25–8	≤2	4	≥8
Gentamicin	1–16	≤4	8	≥16
Neomycin	4–32	b	b	b
Oxytetracycline[a]	0.5–8	≤2	4	≥8
Penicillin	0.12–8	≤0.12		≥0.25
Spectinomycin[a]	8–64	≤32	64	≥128
Sulfadimethoxine	256	≤256		≥512
Tiamulin	0.5–32	≤16		≥32
Tilmicosin[a]	4–64	≤8	16	≥32
Trimethoprim/Sulfamethoxazole	2/38	≤2/38		≥4/76
Tulathromycin[a]	1–64	≤16	32	≥64
Tylosin	0.5–32	b	b	b

[a] Breakpoints based on gram-negative pathogens associated with bovine respiratory disease.
[b] No defined breakpoints.
Data from Angelos JA, Ball LM, Byrne BA. Minimum inhibitory concentrations of selected antimicrobial agents for Moraxella bovoculi associated with infectious bovine keratoconjunctivitis. J Vet Diagn Invest 2011;23:552–5.

the broth microdilution method in 2 studies that evaluated 88 isolates of *Mor bovis* and 57 isolates of *Mor bovoculi*. In **Table 3**, the compiled results from these 2 studies are summarized and show that both *Mor bovis* and *Mor bovoculi* are generally susceptible to a wide variety of antimicrobials. It is important to recognize that there are currently no established veterinary breakpoints approved by the Clinical and Laboratory Standards Institute for use with *Mor bovis* and *Mor bovoculi* isolated from cases of IBK. In this situation, extrapolation from breakpoints established for pathogens associated with bovine respiratory disease can provide guidance when determining an appropriate antibiotic choice. Further information on the use of antibiotic susceptibility testing and extrapolation of results in decision-making for IBK therapy can be found in the article by Lubbers in this issue.

Subconjunctival/Topical Penicillin

Perhaps the most commonly used treatment for IBK is local ocular therapy with penicillin, usually administered in either the bulbar or the palpebral conjunctiva. Two studies have evaluated the levels of penicillin in ocular fluid following subconjunctival injections. A dose of 600,000 IU (2 mL) procaine penicillin injected either through the skin or through the conjunctiva into the subconjunctival space produced a peak penicillin concentration in the conjunctival fluid of approximately 8 IU/mL for either route

Table 3
Compiled data from studies of MIC of *Moraxella bovis* and *Moraxella bovoculi* as determined by the broth microdilution method

	Moraxella bovis		*Moraxella bovoculi*	
Antimicrobial Agent	MIC_{90}	% Resistance	MIC_{90}	% Resistance
Ampicillin	≤0.25	0.0	≤0.25	0.0
Ceftiofur	≤0.12	0.0	≤0.25	0.0
Chlortetracycline	n.t.	n.c.	1	1.8
Clindamycin	n.t.	n.c.	2	3.5
Danofloxacin	n.t.	n.c.	≤0.12	[a]
Enrofloxacin	≤0.06	0.0	≤0.12	1.8
Erythromycin	≤1	0.0	n.t.	n.c.
Florfenicol	≤0.5	n.c.	0.5	3.5
Gentamicin	≤0.5	0.0	≤1	0.0
Lincomycin	≥32	98.8	n.t.	n.c.
Neomycin	n.t.	n.c.	≤4	[a]
Oxytetracycline	≤1.0	0.0	1	3.5
Penicillin	n.t.	n.c.	0.25	12.3
Spectinomycin	≤8.0	n.c.	16	5.3
Sulfadimethoxine	n.t.	n.c.	>256	19.3
Tiamulin	n.t.	n.c.	1	5.3
Tilmicosin	≤1.0	0.0	≤4	3.5
Trimethoprim/Sulfamethoxazole	≤0.25/4.75	0.0	≤2/38	7.0
Tulathromycin	n.t.	n.c.	4	0.0
Tylosin	≤4.0	n.c.	16	[a]

Abbreviations: n.c., not calculated; n.t., not tested.
[a] No defined breakpoints; unable to determine.
Data from Zielinski G, Piscitelli H, Perez-Monti H, et al. Antibiotic sensitivity of an Argentine strain collection of Moraxella bovis. Vet Ther 2000;1:199–204; and Angelos JA, Ball LM, Byrne BA. Minimum inhibitory concentrations of selected antimicrobial agents for Moraxella bovoculi associated with infectious bovine keratoconjunctivitis. J Vet Diagn Invest 2011;23:552–5.

and a duration of therapeutic concentration (DTC; this was defined as 5 times the MIC of penicillin against *Mor bovis*) of approximately 68 hours and approximately 40 hours, respectively.[39] In that study, the difference between the DTCs at these 2 routes were significantly different. When the dose of penicillin was reduced to 1 mL (300,000 IU) given subconjunctivally through the conjunctiva, the DTC was reduced to approximately 35 hours; however, this DTC was not significantly different compared to the DTC from the 2-mL dose given through the conjunctiva. These investigators concluded that all 3 dose routes tested should, in theory, provide adequate anti-*Mor bovis* conjunctival fluid concentrations of penicillin to justify this therapy.

The same investigators also evaluated penicillin concentrations in conjunctival fluid following topical application of sodium benzyl-penicillin, procaine-penicillin, and benethamine-penicillin in various aqueous and ointment bases.[40] The oil-based products produced DTCs that ranged from approximately 37 to approximately 56 hours. In sum, these studies supported a rationale for why the use of penicillin subconjunctivally should be effective, and the study authors suggested that a 48-hour treatment interval should be adequate between penicillin treatments.[39,40]

When penicillin (300,000 U procaine penicillin G; 1 mL) administered either alone or in combination with dexamethasone (1 mL; 4 mg) was dosed subconjunctivally in the superior palpebral conjunctiva once daily for 3 consecutive days, no differences were observed between treatment and untreated control groups in the outcome of naturally occurring IBK.[41] In a subsequent study, when penicillin (300,000 U of procaine penicillin G) was administered subconjunctivally in the bulbar conjunctiva (repeated 48–72 hours later), the prevalence of IBK was significantly reduced among calves that received procaine penicillin G compared with untreated calves in the control group. Most likely the difference in efficacy between these 2 studies can be attributed to differences in the route of penicillin delivery. In the 1995 study, penicillin was administered subconjunctivally in the superior palpebral conjunctiva instead of in the bulbar conconjunctiva.

In a study involving ocular penicillin treatment in dairy cows, a single bulbar subconjunctival dose of procaine penicillin G (300,000 units) resulted in milk penicillin that could be detected for up to 22 hours after injection.[42]

Topical Cloxacillin

Topical ocular application of 250 mg per eye and 375 mg per eye of benzathine cloxacillin was found to be effective against experimentally induced IBK whereby these treatments resulted in lower rates of *Mor bovis* isolations from ocular secretions and reduced clinical scores and corneal ulcer surface areas as compared with control groups of calves.[43] In that study, lower concentrations of benzathine cloxacillin (50 mg per eye and 125 mg per eye) were not found to be effective. In a similar study that evaluated the efficacy of benzathine cloxacillin against naturally occurring IBK, benzathine cloxacillin at the same doses described above was effective, especially when administered early in the course of disease.[44] The commercially available intramammary therapies in the United States that contain cloxacillin deliver between 200 and 500 mg of cloxacillin in a volume of 10 mL. In the studies described above, doses given to calves were contained within a 1-mL volume. The application of 1 mL of an intramammary treatment of a commercially available cloxacillin preparation would only provide a small fraction of the drug levels necessary to achieve the desired doses of cloxacillin that were previously shown to be effective in treating IBK.

Parenteral Oxytetracycline

Compared with untreated calves in the control group, calves that received 2 doses of long-acting oxytetracycline (20 mg/kg; 72 hours apart) had a lower incidence of IBK and decreased duration of *Mor bovis* shedding following experimental infection.[45] This same dose of long-acting oxytetracycline was also found to shorten the number of days of lacrimation and blepharospasm in calves with experimentally induced IBK.[46]

Parenteral Tulathromycin

A single SC dose of tulathromycin (2.5 mg/kg) was compared with no treatment in calves experimentally infected with *Mor bovis*.[47] In that study, the benefits of treatment included significantly fewer isolations of *Mor bovis* from ocular swabs, shorter healing times, lower corneal lesion scores, reduced sizes of corneal ulcers, and development of fewer ulcers bilaterally versus calves in the control group.

Parenteral Florfenicol

Two studies have reported on the efficacy of florfenicol against experimentally induced[48] and naturally occurring IBK.[49] In the experimental study, calves were randomly assigned to receive 2 doses of florfenicol (20 mg/kg IM at 0 and 48 hours), 1 dose of florfenicol (40 mg/kg SC one time), or no treatment (control group). Ulcer healing rates were significantly greater in calves of the IM and SC groups (6.2 and 4.8 times, respectively) versus the control group. Clinical scores and ulcer surface area measurements for the 2 florfenicol groups were significantly lower as compared with the control group. As both IM and SC groups were comparable in most variables evaluated in that study, it was suggested that SC dosing would be advantageous over IM dosing in that there would be decreased tissue damage associated with injections and decreased cost associated with labor with SC treatment. In a study of florfenicol against naturally occurring IBK, corneal ulcer healing rates were significantly greater in the IM and SC groups (3.3 and 2.6 times, respectively) versus the control group, and both routes of administration were considered equally effective.[49]

Parenteral Ceftiofur

The use of ceftiofur crystalline-free acid (CCFA) administered at a single 6.6-mg/kg dose SC in the posterior aspect of the pinna for treatment of corneal ulceration associated with naturally occurring IBK6 was evaluated.[50] In that study, a control group of calves were administered vehicle alone. This treatment resulted in a 4-fold increased odds of corneal ulcer healing by 14 days as compared with calves in the control group and results supported that CCFA was effective against naturally occurring IBK. Although CCFA was shown to be effective against IBK, its use for IBK would be considered extralabel. Since 2012 in the United States, the extralabel uses of cephalosporins (with the exception of approved cephapirin products in food-producing animals) have been prohibited at unapproved dose levels, frequencies, durations, or routes of administration and for disease prevention in cattle, swine, chickens, and turkeys.[35] This US Food and Drug Administration ruling prohibits the use of cephalosporin drugs that are labeled for use in humans or companion animals in cattle if the drug is not approved for use in cattle. Although CCFA could be used to treat IBK, it would have to be dosed exactly according to approved dosing regimens on the product label for specified indications (bovine respiratory disease, foot rot, and acute metritis). Also, according to AMDUCA,[34] the approved antibiotics for treatment of IBK (oxytetracycline and tulathromycin) would have to be determined by a veterinarian working with a client within the context of a valid veterinarian-client-patient relationship to be clinically ineffective in order for ceftiofur to be legally prescribed for use in treatment of IBK.

Parenteral/Intrapalpebral Tilmicosin Versus Intrapalpebral Oxytetracycline

The efficacy of tilmicosin versus no treatment or oxytetracycline was evaluated in one randomized blocked and blinded study.[51] That study evaluated treatment effects over a 21-day period on 120 steers with naturally occurring IBK divided into 6 groups: no treatment (control); oxytetracycline (300 mg intrapalpebral injection; volume not described); tilmicosin (300 mg; 1 mL) administered into the eyelid (intrapalpebral); and tilmicosin administered at 3 different doses (2.5, 5, and 10 mg/kg SC). Results showed that the percentage improvement in clinical signs (ocular discharge, blepharospasm, and corneal lesion scores—a measurement that took into account the severity of corneal opacity, ulceration, vision compromise, and presence of globe rupture) between day 0 and 21 were significantly higher for the 10 mg/kg SC tilmicosin group versus the control and oxytetracycline group. Significantly higher percentage improvement in corneal lesion scores from day 0 to day 21 was observed in the tilmicosin treatment groups versus the oxytetracycline group, but not between the control versus tilmicosin treatment groups. The study authors concluded that tilmicosin at

5 or 10 mg/kg SC was therapeutically beneficial; however, they did not recommend use of tilmicosin by the intrapalpebral route.

Parenteral Florfenicol Versus Parenteral Oxytetracycline

One randomized study compared the efficacy of florfenicol versus oxytetracycline (each drug dosed at 20 mg/kg IM; 2 doses 48 hours apart) in 30 Brown Swiss calves with naturally occurring IBK over a 10-week period; in this study, blinding of study personnel was not described.[26] The results of the study reported that although photophobia and lacrimation decreased only slightly at 48 hours in the oxytetracycline-treated group, these signs disappeared completely at 24 hours in the florfenicol group. The mean time to disappearance of corneal opacity was 13.14 ± 3.39 days in the florfenicol group versus 18.56 ± 6.18 days in 9 of 15 calves in the oxytetracycline group. IBK reoccurred in 3 of 15 oxytetracycline-treated calves during weeks 6 and 7 of the follow-up period; however, no reoccurrences were observed in the florfenicol-treated calves. The overall conclusion of the study authors was that florfenicol was more effective than oxytetracycline. Whether these conclusions are justified is difficult to determine because there were limited study data available in the results and no reported results of any statistical analysis.

Parenteral Plus Oral Oxytetracycline Versus Subconjunctival Penicillin

The use of combined oral plus parenteral (SC) oxytetracycline to ameliorate IBK during an outbreak was evaluated in 119 Hereford calves.[52] In that study, calves were randomly assigned to receive either no treatment (control group), 300,000 U of procaine penicillin G subconjunctivally in the bulbar conjunctiva (repeated 48–72 hours later), or a combined parenteral plus oral oxytetracycline treatment. In the oxytetracycline group, calves were administered an injection of a long-acting formulation of oxytetracycline (20 mg/kg IM; repeated again 72 hours later if ulcers were present on days 1 and 2) plus oral oxytetracycline (2 g per calf per day) for 10 days delivered in alfalfa pellets. Calves were examined 3 times per week for 7 weeks. Calves in the oxytetracycline group had significantly fewer ulcer recurrences versus control or penicillin group calves. The oxytetracycline group also had a significantly lower prevalence of IBK versus control group and penicillin group calves during days 11 through 49 and 21 through 49, respectively. *Moraxella bovis* was isolated from significantly fewer ocular secretion specimens from calves in the oxytetracycline group versus either the control or the penicillin-treated groups. Between days 1 to 10 and 40 to 49, *Moraxella bovis* was isolated from significantly fewer ocular secretion specimens from calves in the penicillin group versus calves in the control group. Corneal ulcer healing times were significantly lower for both the oxytetracycline and the penicillin treatment groups versus the control group. The authors of this study concluded that both oxytetracycline and penicillin (injected subconjunctivally in the bulbar conjunctiva) were effective in reducing healing times of corneal ulcers associated with IBK. The reduced prevalence of IBK as well as the reduced number of calves developing recurrent ulcers in the oxytetracycline group versus the penicillin group suggested that oxytetracycline treatment was superior to penicillin treatment. It is not known, however, whether the benefit of oxytetracycline was attributable to parenteral treatment, oral treatment, or both from this study; however, another study had previously demonstrated the benefit of parenteral oxytetracycline (2 doses of 20 mg/kg IM 72 hours apart) in reducing the incidence of IBK and decreasing the duration of *Mor bovis* shedding.[45] It is important to remember that under current federal laws in the United States, use of oxytetracycline in feed to treat IBK would be illegal because extralabel use of drugs in animal feed is prohibited.[35]

Intrapalpebral Versus Parenteral Oxytetracycline

Oxytetracycline administered by the intrapalpebral (200 mg oxytetracycline hydro-chloride solution [10%] injected through the skin) versus IM (20 mg/kg) routes was evaluated for the treatment of calves with naturally occurring IBK.[53] In this study, both treatments were similar in the mean number of treatments per animal and the interval between diagnosis and healing; however, significantly less medication was required for the intrapalpebral group. As expected, the calves with intrapalpebral injections of oxytetracycline developed large swellings around the eye that disappeared by 72 hours after injection. Although administration of oxytetracycline intrapalpebrally through the skin was considered effective, the administration of long-acting oxytetracycline (100 mg in the bulbar conjunctiva), however, was found in another study to cause conjunctival chemosis and necrosis and was not recommended.[54]

Other Pharmacologic Treatment Options

Antibiotic therapy for acute cases of IBK is generally recommended; however, no generally accepted guidelines exist on when to treat versus not treat based on corneal ulcer size. In the author's experience, ulcers that are less than 5 mm maximal diameter will often heal spontaneously; however, this is not always the case and in valuable animals or where concerns exist for an outbreak, antibiotics are recommended. In developing standard operating procedures for the treatment of IBK for owners, it is important to emphasize that every calf with a cloudy-appearing eye does not necessarily require antibiotics. For example, a calf with the eye shown in **Fig. 9** has a cloudy eye; however, further antibiotic treatment of this animal is not necessary, because the ulcer is healed and blood vessels are covering the entire lesion. In the author's experience, it is useful to give clients photographs of healed and unhealed eyes to educate them on how to identify corneal neovascularization. When corneal neovascularization has bridged the corneal defect, antibiotics are not usually necessary.

Besides antibiotics, treatment with a nonsteroidal anti-inflammatory drug, such as flunixin meglumine, is likely to reduce ocular inflammation and improve the comfort level of the animal. Use of other drugs such as atropine could be considered; however, titrating atropine treatment to effect can be impractical in field settings.

The addition of dexamethasone (1 mL; 4 mg) to penicillin (300,000 U) administered in the superior palpebral conjunctiva did not appear to alter corneal ulcer healing time, severity, diameter, surface area measurement, or frequency of ulcer recurrence versus untreated calves or calves treated with penicillin alone.[41]

One of the older treatments that cattle producers sometimes mention as being extremely effective is the use of "puffers" that deliver nitrofurazone topically in the eye. Although this treatment is effective, nitrofurazone is strictly prohibited from extra-label use in food-producing animals in the United States.[55] Because there are currently no nitrofurazone-containing products that carry any label approval for use in food-producing animals, this prohibition effectively bans any use of nitrofurazone products in food animals. This prohibition also applies to any remaining older products that may have indicated approval for use in cattle for treatment of IBK.

NONPHARMACOLOGIC TREATMENT OPTIONS

In more intensive treatment settings, application of autologous patient serum eye drops harvested from whole blood can provide corneal growth factors and anticollagenase activities that may aid in corneal ulcer healing.[56] In field settings, this therapy is usually impractical because frequent (every 30–60 minutes) dosing is probably necessary to provide the most benefit. Dosing as often as is practically possible, however, should not be harmful and may be practical under some field settings with dedicated owners. To prepare serum, it should be harvested under as sterile conditions as possible and then maintained under refrigeration and replaced every few days.

The use of denim patches to cover eyes of cattle with IBK can provide comfort to an affected animal by reducing ambient light and can also reduce exposure of flies to ocular secretions, which can harbor *Moraxella* spp. When advising owners on use and application of patches, it is a good idea to recommend that a ventral opening be left to prevent build-up of ocular secretions and humidity and to remind owners to check eyes frequently after patches are placed to make sure that ulcers are not worsening under the patch.

Although no studies have evaluated ocular healing of trace mineral deficient and trace mineral replete cattle with experimentally induced IBK, it is likely that adequate trace mineral status (often copper and selenium) is important in maintaining optimal immune responses in cattle at risk of developing or that have already developed IBK.

Moraxella bovis is known to survive in and on flies,[23–26] and reducing fly burden is an extremely important part of any IBK control program. A variety of different fly control products and methods of delivery are available, and a complete listing of all such products is beyond the scope of this discussion. For further information on the availability of such products, consultations with local, county, and agriculture extension agents may be informative. If producers are using insecticide-impregnated ear tags, it is important to stress that such ear tags should be placed on (at the very least) calves and should be removed at the end of the fly season to prevent the development of insecticide resistance.

COMBINATION THERAPIES

The use of multiple antibiotics in the treatment of IBK under field settings is not generally recommended for economic reasons as well as from the standpoint of good stewardship relative to antibiotic use and concerns over the development of antimicrobial resistance. *Moraxella bovis* and *Mor bovoculi* are typically very sensitive organisms and should respond to appropriate single-drug therapies. In cases where multiple organisms (for example, *Mycoplasma* spp plus Moraxellae) may be responsible for ongoing disease in a herd, it is important to select an appropriate antibiotic class that would be effective against both types of organisms. Tulathromycin is currently licensed to treat IBK in the United States and also has a label claim for treatment and control of respiratory disease associated with *Mycoplasma bovis*. Whether this drug would be effective under field settings in controlling an IBK outbreak that involves *Mycoplasma* spp is not known. In cases where the involvement of *Mycoplasma* spp is being considered, it is also important to remember that the use of a β-lactam antibiotic (eg, penicillin or a cephalosporin class drug) that kills by inhibiting cell wall synthesis would be ineffective against an organism such as mycoplasma that lacks a cell wall.

SURGICAL TREATMENT OPTIONS

Surgical treatment options that have been used in treating cattle with IBK include third eyelid flaps and tarsorrhaphy. In cases in which globe rupture has occurred or where severe scar formation and globe protrusion represents a potential liability to the animal, exenteration may be indicated.

TREATMENT RESISTANCE/COMPLICATIONS

For an individual animal, a treatment failure should be considered when the severity of corneal ulceration is worsening or other clinical signs related to IBK are not improving. When therapy is delayed, corneal scarring can lead to reduced vision and possibly globe rupture and permanent blindness. At the herd level, failure of a pinkeye treatment and control program is apparent when numbers of active cases are observed to be increasing over time. When a specific antibiotic treatment does not appear to be working, it is worth collecting ocular samples for bacterial culture and sensitivity testing. Samples should be collected from animals with early cases that have not been treated. Collecting samples from as many affected animals as possible is recommended, ideally from 10% to 20% of affected animals. Testing on such a scale can be cost prohibitive, however, and at the very least it is recommended that samples be collected from 10 to 12 animals if possible. As mentioned above, it can be cost saving to contact the clinical microbiology laboratory before sample collection to make sure that appropriate samples in the correct media are submitted along with an accurate culture request. If the development of an autogenous bacterin is being considered by your client, it is valuable to request that the laboratory preserve isolates for future use and submission to a vaccine manufacturer.

EVALUATION OF OUTCOME AND LONG-TERM RECOMMENDATIONS

With successful therapy, an IBK-affected animal will generally seem more comfortable with reduced ocular discharge and improved ability to hold open the eyelids. In outbreak or potential outbreak situations, early recognition of treatment failures is important and should prompt a discussion with the client or herd manager on a variety of topics that cover issues such as how the treatments are being done, whether gloves are being worn, and if equipment is being disinfected between animals. When vaccines are being used, it is important to stress the importance of proper timing of vaccination relative to when IBK typically occurs in a herd. Although there are widely divergent views on the merits of vaccination for IBK, producers who use vaccines should recognize that the full potential to realize a vaccine benefit is optimized when a vaccine series is initiated at least 4 weeks before the typical IBK season. In any herd setting, IBK is never just an individual animal problem, and identification of IBK should prompt discussions with producers on all aspects of IBK control and prevention, including reduction of potential risk factors for disease (flies, foreign bodies [plant awns, dust], ultraviolet radiation, concurrent infections [*Mycoplasma* spp, IBR, possibly *Mor bovoculi*]), vaccinations, and trace mineral status and supplementation.

SUMMARY

As is the case for controlling other infectious livestock diseases, the most successful efforts to control IBK will include consideration of multiple facets of disease control, including the host, the environment, herd management, and ongoing surveillance even after the immediate crisis has passed. Research over a period of many years has led to the discovery of a variety of antibiotic treatments and antibiotic regimens that can be effective against IBK. The discoveries of *Mor bovoculi* and reports of IBK associated with *Mycoplasma* spp without concurrent *Mor bovis* or *Mor bovoculi* have raised new questions into the roles that other organisms may play in IBK. When collecting samples for submission to clinical microbiology laboratories, patient selection and correct sample submission are vitally important to maximize the chances for obtaining useful information. Discussions of IBK control programs with producers should take into consideration all aspects of the disease, including the host immune response and reduction of potential risk factors.

SUPPLEMENTARY DATA

Supplementary data related to this article can be found online at http://dx.doi.org/10.1016/j.cvfa.2014.11.006.

REFERENCES

1. Frisch JE. The relative incidence and effect of bovine infectious keratoconjunctivitis in Bos indicus and Bos taurus cattle. Anim Prod 1975;21:265–74.
2. Snowder GD, Van Vleck LD, Cundiff LV, et al. Genetic and environmental factors associated with incidence of infectious bovine keratoconjunctivitis in preweaned beef calves. J Anim Sci 2005;83:507–18.
3. Webber JJ, Selby LA. Risk factors related to the prevalence of infectious bovine keratoconjunctivitis. J Am Vet Med Assoc 1981;179:823–6.
4. Ward JK, Neilson MK. Pinkeye (bovine infectious keratoconjunctivitis) in beef cattle. J Anim Sci 1979;49:361–6.
5. Jayappa HG, Lehr C. Pathogenicity and immunogenicity of piliated and nonpiliated phases of Moraxella bovis in calves. Am J Vet Res 1986;47:2217–21.
6. Annuar BO, Wilcox GE. Adherence of Moraxella bovis to cell cultures of bovine origin. Res Vet Sci 1985;39:241–6.
7. Hoien-Dalen PS, Rosenbusch RF, Roth JA. Comparative characterization of the leukocidic and hemolytic activity of Moraxella bovis. Am J Vet Res 1990;51: 191–6.
8. Kagonyera GM, George LW, Munn R. Cytopathic effects of Moraxella bovis on cultured bovine neutrophils and corneal epithelial cells. Am J Vet Res 1989;50: 10–7.
9. Kagonyera GM, George LW, Munn R. Light and electron microscopic changes in corneas of healthy and immunomodulated calves infected with Moraxella bovis. Am J Vet Res 1988;49:386–95.
10. Rogers DG, Cheville NF, Pugh GW Jr. Pathogenesis of corneal lesions caused by Moraxella bovis in gnotobiotic calves. Vet Pathol 1987;24:287–95.
11. Angelos JA, Spinks PQ, Ball LM, et al. Moraxella bovoculi sp. nov., isolated from calves with infectious bovine keratoconjunctivitis. Int J Syst Evol Microbiol 2007; 57:789–95.
12. Gould S, Dewell R, Tofflemire K, et al. Randomized blinded challenge study to assess association between Moraxella bovoculi and infectious bovine keratoconjunctivitis in dairy calves. Vet Microbiol 2013;164:108–15.
13. Angelos JA, Ball LM, Hess JF. Identification and characterization of complete RTX operons in Moraxella bovoculi and Moraxella ovis. Vet Microbiol 2007;125:73–9.
14. Calcutt MJ, Foecking MF, Martin NT, et al. Draft genome sequence of Moraxella bovoculi strain 237T (ATCC BAA-1259T) isolated from a calf with infectious bovine keratoconjunctivitis. Genome Announc 2014;2(3).
15. George LW, Ardans A, Mihalyi J, et al. Enhancement of infectious bovine keratoconjunctivitis by modified-live infectious bovine rhinotracheitis virus vaccine. Am J Vet Res 1988;49:1800–6.
16. Pugh GW Jr, Hughes DE, Packer RA. Bovine infectious keratoconjunctivitis: interactions of Moraxella bovis and infectious bovine rhinotracheitis virus. Am J Vet Res 1970;31:653–62.

17. Pugh GW, Hughes DE, Schulz VD. Infectious bovine keratoconjunctivitis: experimental induction of infection in calves with mycoplasmas and Moraxella bovis. Am J Vet Res 1976;37:493–5.
18. Rosenbusch RF. Influence of mycoplasma preinfection on the expression of Moraxella bovis pathogenicity. Am J Vet Res 1983;44:1621–4.
19. Lepper AW, Barton IJ. Infectious bovine keratoconjunctivitis: seasonal variation in cultural, biochemical and immunoreactive properties of Moraxella bovis isolated from the eyes of cattle. Aust Vet J 1987;64:33–9.
20. Pugh GW, McDonald TJ, Kopecky KE. Infectious bovine keratoconjunctivitis: effects of vaccination on Moraxella bovis carrier state in cattle. Am J Vet Res 1980; 41:264–6.
21. Hughes DE, Pugh GW Jr, McDonald TJ. Ultraviolet radiation and Moraxella bovis in the etiology of bovine infectious keratoconjunctivitis. Am J Vet Res 1965;26: 1331–8.
22. Hughes DE, Pugh GW, McDonald TJ. Experimental bovine infectious keratoconjunctivitis caused by sunlamp irradiation and Moraxella bovis infection: resistance to re-exposure with homologous and heterologous Moraxella bovis. Am J Vet Res 1968;29:829–33.
23. Arends JJ, Wright RE, Barto PB, et al. Transmission of Moraxella bovis from blood agar cultures to Hereford cattle by face flies (Diptera: Muscidae). J Econ Entomol 1984;77:394–8.
24. Glass HW Jr, Gerhardt RR, Greene WH. Survival of Moraxella bovis in the alimentary tract of the face fly. J Econ Entomol 1982;75:545–6.
25. Steve PC, Lilly JH. Investigations on transmissability of Moraxella bovis by the face fly. J Econ Entomol 1965;58:444–6.
26. Gokce HI, Citil M, Genc O, et al. A comparison of the efficacy of florfenicol and oxytetracycline in the treatment of naturally occurring infectious bovine keratoconjunctivitis. Irish Vet J 2002;55:573–6.
27. Naglic T, Sankovic F, Madic J, et al. Mycoplasmas associated with bovine conjunctivitis and keratoconjunctivitis. Acta Vet Hung 1996;44:21–4.
28. Levisohn S, Garazi S, Gerchman I, et al. Diagnosis of a mixed mycoplasma infection associated with a severe outbreak of bovine pinkeye in young calves. J Vet Diagn Invest 2004;16:579–81.
29. Alberti A, Addis MF, Chessa B, et al. Molecular and antigenic characterization of a Mycoplasma bovis strain causing an outbreak of infectious keratoconjunctivitis. J Vet Diagn Invest 2006;18:41–51.
30. Funk LD, Reecy JM, Wang C, et al. Associations between infectious bovine keratoconjunctivitis at weaning and ultrasonographically measured body composition traits in yearling cattle. J Am Vet Med Assoc 2014;244:100–6.
31. Killinger AH, Valentine D, Mansfield ME, et al. Economic impact of infectious bovine keratoconjunctivitis in beef calves. Vet Med Small Anim Clin 1977;72:618–20.
32. Thrift FA, Overfield JR. Impact of pinkeye (infectious bovine kerato-conjunctivitis) on weaning and postweaning performance of Hereford calves. J Anim Sci 1974; 38:1179–84.
33. O'Connor AM, Wellman NG, Evans RB, et al. A review of randomized clinical trials reporting antibiotic treatment of infectious bovine keratoconjunctivitis in cattle. Anim Health Res Rev 2006;7:119–27.
34. Animal Medicinal Drug Use Clarification Act of 1994 (AMDUCA). U.S. Food and Drug Administration. Available at: http://www.fda.gov/AnimalVeterinary/GuidanceComplianceEnforcement/ActsRulesRegulations/ucm085377.htm. Accessed August 31, 2014.

35. CFR - Code of Federal Regulations Title 21. U.S. Food and Drug Administration. Available at: http://www.accessdata.fda.gov/scripts/cdrh/cfdocs/cfcfr/CFRSearch.cfm?CFRPart=530. Accessed August 31, 2014.

36. Chandler RL, Smith K, Turfrey BA. Ultrastructural and histological studies on the corneal lesion in infectious bovine keratoconjunctivitis. J Comp Pathol 1981;91: 175–84.

37. Zielinski G, Piscitelli H, Perez-Monti H, et al. Antibiotic sensitivity of an Argentine strain collection of Moraxella bovis. Vet Ther 2000;1:199–204.

38. Angelos JA, Ball LM, Byrne BA. Minimum inhibitory concentrations of selected antimicrobial agents for Moraxella bovoculi associated with infectious bovine keratoconjunctivitis. J Vet Diagn Invest 2011;23:552–5.

39. Abeynayake P, Cooper BS. The concentration of penicillin in bovine conjunctival sac fluid as it pertains to the treatment of Moraxella bovis infection. (I) Subconjunctival injection. J Vet Pharmacol Ther 1989;12:25–30.

40. Abeynayake P, Cooper BS. The concentration of penicillin in bovine conjunctival sac fluid as it pertains to the treatment of Moraxella bovis infection. (II) Topical application. J Vet Pharmacol Ther 1989;12:31–6.

41. Allen LJ, George LW, Willits NH. Effect of penicillin or penicillin and dexamethasone in cattle with infectious bovine keratoconjunctivitis. J Am Vet Med Assoc 1995;206:1200–3.

42. Liljebjelke KA, Warnick LD, Witt MF. Antibiotic residues in milk following bulbar subconjunctival injection of procaine penicillin G in dairy cows. J Am Vet Med Assoc 2000;217:369–71.

43. Daigneault J, George LW. Topically applied benzathine cloxacillin for treatment of experimentally induced infectious bovine keratoconjunctivitis. Am J Vet Res 1990; 51:376–80.

44. George LW, Keefe T, Daigneault J. Effectiveness of two benzathine cloxacillin formulations for treatment of naturally occurring infectious bovine keratoconjunctivitis. Am J Vet Res 1989;50:1170–4.

45. George LW, Smith JA. Treatment of Moraxella bovis infections in calves using a long-acting oxytetracycline formulation. J Vet Pharmacol Ther 1985;8:55–61.

46. Smith JA, George LW. Treatment of acute ocular Moraxella bovis infections in calves with a parenterally administered long-acting oxytetracycline formulation. Am J Vet Res 1985;46:804–7.

47. Lane VM, George LW, Cleaver DM. Efficacy of tulathromycin for treatment of cattle with acute ocular Moraxella bovis infections. J Am Vet Med Assoc 2006;229:557–61.

48. Dueger EL, Angelos JA, Cosgrove S, et al. Efficacy of florfenicol in the treatment of experimentally induced infectious bovine keratoconjunctivitis. Am J Vet Res 1999;60:960–4.

49. Angelos JA, Dueger EL, George LW, et al. Efficacy of florfenicol for treatment of naturally occurring infectious bovine keratoconjunctivitis. J Am Vet Med Assoc 2000;216:62–4.

50. Dueger EL, George LW, Angelos JA, et al. Efficacy of a long-acting formulation of ceftiofur crystalline-free acid for the treatment of naturally occurring infectious bovine keratoconjunctivitis. Am J Vet Res 2004;65:1185–8.

51. Zielinski GC, Piscitelli HG, Perez-Monti H, et al. Efficacy of different dosage levels and administration routes of tilmicosin in a natural outbreak of infectious bovine keratoconjunctivitis (pinkeye). Vet Ther 2002;3:196–205.

52. Eastman TG, George LW, Hird DW, et al. Combined parenteral and oral administration of oxytetracycline for control of infectious bovine keratoconjunctivitis. J Am Vet Med Assoc 1998;212:560–3.

53. Starke A, Eule C, Meyer H, et al. Efficacy of intrapalpebral and intramuscular application of oxytetracycline in a natural outbreak of infectious bovine kertoconjunctivitis (IBK) in calves. Dtsch Tierarztl Wochenschr 2007;114:219–24.
54. George LW, Wilson WD, Baggot JD, et al. Antibiotic treatment of Moraxella bovis infection in cattle. J Am Vet Med Assoc 1984;185:1206–9.
55. Electronic Code of Federal Regulations. Title 21: Food and Drugs. Part 530-Extralabel Drug Use in Animals. Available at: http://www.ecfr.gov/cgi-bin/text-idx?SID= 054808d261de27898e02fb175b7c9ff9&node=21:6.0.1.1.16&rgn=div5#se21.6.530_ 141. Accessed September 1, 2014.
56. Maggs DJ, Miller PE, Ofri R. Slatter's fundamentals of veterinary ophthalmology. 4th edition. St Louis (MO): Saunders Elsevier; 2008. p. 189.

Clinical Evidence for Individual Animal Therapy for Papillomatous Digital Dermatitis (Hairy Heel Wart) and Infectious Bovine Pododermatitis (Foot Rot)

CrossMark

Michael D. Apley, DVM, PhD

KEYWORDS

- Papillomatous digital dermatitis • Hairy heel wart • Infectious bovine podoermatitis
- Foot rot • Interdigital necrobacillosis • Therapy • Clinical trials
- Susceptibility testing

KEY POINTS

- Clinical evidence presented here was limited to randomized, prospective clinical trials conducted in naturally occurring disease with negative controls and masked subjective evaluators.
- In the case of papillomatous digital dermatitis (PDD), these trials support the use of topical tetracycline and oxytetracycline, lincomycin, a copper-containing preparation, and a non-antimicrobial cream; there is a significant effect of stage of disease on treatment success as measured by disease recurrence.
- Susceptibility testing of *Treponema* spp isolates and parallels with *Treponema*-associated disease in humans supports the potential for systemic use of macrolides and some β-lactams, but clinical trial confirmation is needed.
- In the case of individual therapy for infectious pododermatitis (IP), trial evidence is available to support systemic treatment with ceftiofur, florfenicol, tulathromycin, and oxytetracycline; clinical trial evidence was not readily available for common IP therapies such as penicillin G, sulfadimethoxine, and tylosin.

Author Disclosures: Author has accepted research funding and consulting fees from Zoetis (maker of cefitofur, a penicillin G, tulathromycin, lincomycin, and an oxytetracycline), Elanco (maker of tylosin), and Merial (maker of gamithromycinfor).
Department of Clinical Sciences, Kansas State University College of Veterinary Medicine, 1800 Denison Avenue, Manhattan, KS 66506, USA
E-mail address: mapley@vet.ksu.edu

INTRODUCTION

The use of drugs to treat infectious disease, especially antimicrobials, is based on the clinician's judgment that the drug will make a difference in clinical outcome in a population over time. Clinical trial reports are the pinnacle of evidence to support this judgment, followed by physiologic reasoning such as antimicrobial susceptibility testing combined with antimicrobial pharmacokinetic and pharmacodynamic characteristics. This article evaluates clinical trial and supportive data to inform clinician decisions on individual animal treatment of 2 common infectious diseases of the bovine foot.

To be included in the evidence tables of this article, clinical trials must have met the following criteria:

- Prospective
- Randomized
- Naturally occurring disease
- Negative controls
- Masking of subjective evaluators

Strict adherence to these requirements may have eliminated some studies that met these criteria, but for which reporting was incomplete. These situations underscore the importance of adhering to reporting guidelines such as the reporting guidelines for randomized controlled trials in livestock and food safety (REFLECT) statement, which are also helpful in study design in anticipation of successful publication.[1] In particular, the requirement for masking of subjective evaluators eliminated several publications. Another observation is that investigators are well advised to consult statisticians during study design and to clarify the appropriate analysis and reporting of categorical data such as clinical scores.

The outcomes of the clinical trials were summarized and then characterized in the form of the number needed to treat (NNT) statistic.[2] The NNT is calculated by first determining the absolute risk reduction (ARR), which is the actual difference in percentage clinical success between the treated and negative control groups. The ARR is then divided into 100%, with the resulting value representing the NNT; this is the number of animals that must be treated to make a difference in 1 animal. Because the NNT is based on the difference between treated and untreated animals in the same diseased population, it represents the effect of the drug in consideration of the spontaneous cure rate of the population, which in turn gives some insight into the severity of the disease challenge. Comparison of NNT values is only valid within the same study; comparing NNT values between studies to determine the most effective drug is inappropriate because of the potential differences in the disease challenge.

The external relevance of these trials is affected by the case definitions and the time of detection of disease in relation to field applications. An attempt has been made to describe case definitions, but the reader is directed to the original articles for more detail so that external relevance of the data may be further evaluated.

PAPILLOMATOUS DIGITAL DERMATITIS (HAIRY HEEL WART, STRAWBERRY FOOT ROT)

The therapy of PDD still lacks clarity as to the breadth of etiologic agents and pathogenesis. The multifactorial cause has been documented in the literature, with a consistent finding of spirochete organisms of the genus *Treponema* as well as multiple genera and species of bacteria.[3–8]

Available clinical trials for individual animal therapy that met inclusion criteria for evidence tables were limited to topical therapy. No reports of systemic therapy for

PDD met inclusion criteria. There is substantial literature on the use of foot baths for control of PDD, which is not addressed here.[9–17]

Randomized, Masked, Prospective Trials with Negative Controls for Topical Therapy for Papillomatous Digital Dermatitis

Four studies involving PDD were identified and are summarized in **Table 1**. Study entry case definitions and success/failure definitions applied at the end of the study period are presented in the table. As with all clinical trials, these definitions have an effect on the external validity of the studies in relation to applicability in a practice setting.

Cutler and colleagues[18] conducted a study in an Ontario dairy wherein 214 hooves were treated with tetracycline HCl powder (2–5 g) under a bandage for 2 days or a prepared tetracycline HCl paste (2–5 g) with no bandage, or were not treated. Cows that were severely lame were only assigned to one of the positive treatment groups because of welfare concerns. As part of the preventive program on the farm, all cattle walked through a foot bath 3 times a week regardless of the study status; the foot bath treatments were copper sulfate (58 g/L) twice weekly and tetracycline (1.16 g/L) once weekly. At 8 to 12 days posttreatment, healing rates were 57.1% in the tetracycline

Table 1
Evidence from randomized, masked, prospective clinical trials for individual animal therapy for papillomatous digital dermatitis expressed as percentage success and NNT

Case Definition	Success Definition	N	Treatments	% with Positive Case Outcome	NNT
Raw, moist lesions with tufted or granular surfaces as scored by investigator	Lesion healing at 8–12 d posttreatment (no sign of moist surface or scab)	65	Untreated control	0.0%	___
		70	Tetracycline HCl powder with bandage for 2 d	57.1%	1.75 (2)
		79	Tetracycline HCl paste once	47.4%	2.11 (2)
Active, red digital dermatitis lesion	Decision not to retreat at 29 d—based on signs of pain, lesion activity, or both	33	Untreated control	3.1%	___
		33	Lincomycin paste	93.7%	1.10 (1)
		32	Nonantimicrobial cream	69.7%	1.50 (2)
Lesion with signs of severe pain	The reference reports pain and lesion scores at days 14 and 30. For this table, presence of pain at day 30 is reported	10	Control: tap water	20.0%	___
		11	Oxytetracycline solution	80.0%	1.67 (2)
		14	Copper, peroxide, cationic agent	78.6%	1.71 (2)
		10	5% copper sulfate	20.0%	___
		11	Acidified ionized copper solution	0.0%	___
		10	Hydrogen peroxide-peroxyacetic acid	0.0%	___
Pain with visually active lesion, also confirmed histologically	Healed based on assignment of a visual lesion score at 30 d	3	Control, bandage only	0.0%	___
		11	Lincomycin paste (10 g)	72.7%	1.38 (1)
		11	Oxytetracycline paste (10 g)	63.6%	1.57 (2)

Data from Refs.[18–21]

powder hooves, 57.4% in the tetracycline paste hooves, and zero in the negative controls.

Moore and colleagues[19] evaluated the efficacy of lincomycin paste (10 g lincomycin and 3 mL deionized water as a paste) or a nonantimicrobial cream (soluble copper with peroxide and a cationic agent [Victory foot cream]), against negative controls in 98 dairy cows. The products were placed on a 4×4-in gauze sponge (similar volumes) and held in place on the lesion with an elastic bandage for 5 days, after which they were removed by farm personnel. A success or failure definition based on the signs of pain, lesion activity, or both was applied at 29 days, after which the failures would receive re-treatment with the same compound and negative controls would be allocated to one of the treatment compounds. Success rates for the lincomycin, nonantimicrobial cream, and controls were 93.7%, 69.7%, and 3.1%, respectively. All treatments were statistically significant in their differences from the control group with regard to lack of re-treatment. When compared with negative controls, the investigators calculated that cattle treated with lincomycin paste were 31 times more likely to not be re-treated and that the cattle treated with the nonantimicrobial cream were 22.3 times more likely to be not re-treated.

Hernandez and colleagues evaluated 5 topical treatments against a negative control.[20] The treatments were (1) oxytetracycline soluble powder mixed at 25 mg/ml (Terramycin soluble powder, Pfizer Animal Health, Exton, PA); (2) a commercial formulation of soluble copper, peroxide compound, and a cationic agent (Victory, Babson Bros Co., Romeoville, IL); (3) 5% copper sulfate solution, (4) acidified ionized copper solution, (5) hydrogen peroxide-peroxyacetic acid (HPPA) solution (Hoof Pro Plus, SSI Corporation, Julesburg, CO), and (6) tap water negative control. Cows were enrolled with lesions involving a single hind foot which displayed pain categorized as severe. Treatments were applied daily by spray bottle for 5 days, no treatment was applied for 2 days, then treatments were applied every other day for three additional applications. Treatments 1 and 2 were significantly different from the other 4 based on pain at days 14 and 30, and based on visible lesions at day 30. On day 14, treatments 1 and 2 were not significantly different from each other based on visible lesions, but treatment 2 was also not significantly different from treatments 3 and 4. The results of this study summarized by treatment are presented in **Table 1**.

Berry and colleagues[21] treated affected cattle with either lincomycin powder, 10 g, or oxytetracycline powder, 10 g, both mixed with sufficient water to create a paste. Bandages were left on for 4 days. On initial examination, both lesion identification and demonstration of pain were required to be enrolled in the study. The low number of controls[3] was justified by minimizing untreated cattle in a commercial dairy, and response rates of both treated and untreated cattle are similar to those in other studies reported here. The response rates were not significantly different between the positive treatments, 72.7% and 63.6% in the lincomycin and oxytetracycline groups, respectively. This response rate was determined from visual evaluation of lesion healing. Unique to this study, the investigators also evaluated histologic samples from the lesions. Of the 15 lesions classified as healed on study day 30, 7 were still classified as active histologically and 5 were classified as in early stages of development. Histology could not determine if these lesions represented incomplete healing or the initial stages of reinfection. This fact speaks to the concerns about the common recurrence of disease in cattle initially classified as healed. This study also evaluated the microbiology of the lesions, confirming the presence of spirochetes and multiple bacterial species, most of which were not present in control skin cultures from nondiseased cattle. In another study, Berry and colleagues[22] documented that variation in the type of lesion at treatment correlated with the odds of being a healed lesion at the end of the 341-day study. These results emphasize the impact of lesion type on treatment success and disease recurrence and that prognosis and treatment strategies should be affected by lesion characterization.

In vitro Susceptibility Testing of Papillomatous Digital Dermatitis Treponema Isolates

Two publications have evaluated in vitro susceptibility of treponemes isolated from bovine PDD.[23,24] These results are presented in **Table 2**, with comparison to approved

Table 2
MIC_{90} and MBC_{90} for *Treponema* isolates as related to CLSI veterinary breakpoints for other diseases expressed as MIC

DA2:D20	MIC_{90} (μg/mL)	MBC_{90} (μg/mL)	CLSI Veterinary Breakpoints for Other Diseases (μg/mL)
Evans, 2009 (16 isolates from UK cattle, 3 from an ovine outbreak)			
Ampicillin	0.38	1.5	0.25[a]
Enrofloxacin[b]	96	192	0.25[c]
Erythromycin	0.05	0.19	0.5[d]
Gentamicin	24	96	2[e]
Lincomycin	24	48	0.5[f]
Oxytetracycline	0.75	6	2[c]
Penicillin	0.05	0.19	0.25[c]
Spectinomycin	12	48	32[c]
Evans, 2012 (12 isolates from the United Kingdom)			
Amoxicillin	0.38	1.5	0.25[a]
Azithromycin	0.05	0.09	___
Cefalexin	48	192	2[g]
Ceftiofur	6	24	2[c]
Gamithromycin	0.02	0.09	4[h]
Ciprofloxacin[b,i]	48	96	0.25[c]
Colistin[i]	>384	>384	___
Trimethoprim[i]	192	384	___

Abbreviation: CLSI, Clinical and Laboratory Standards Institute.

[a] CLSI susceptible breakpoint for canine skin and soft tissue and equine respiratory disease. The swine respiratory breakpoint is 0.5.

[b] Both of these fluoroquinolones would be illegal for this extralabel use in the United States and some other countries.

[c] CLSI susceptible breakpoint for bovine respiratory disease for ceftiofur, enrofloxacin, gamithromycin, oxytetracycline, penicillin, and spectinomycin.

[d] CLSI susceptible breakpoint for *Entercoccus* spp and *Streptococcus* spp. adapted from human medicine.

[e] CLSI susceptible breakpoints for specific organisms in canine and equine systemic disease.

[f] CLSI susceptible breakpoint for clindamycin in canine skin and soft tissue disease.

[g] CLSI susceptible breakpoint for cephalothin in canine diseases and cefazolin in canine and equine diseases.

[h] CLSI susceptible breakpoint for bovine respiratory disease, approved to come out in next CLSI table edition.

[i] Evaluated for use in *Treponema* isolation media.

Data from CLSI. VET01-S2 performance standards for antimicrobial disk and dilution susceptibility tests for bacteria isolated from animals: second informational supplement. Wayne (PA): Clinical and Laboratory Standards Institute; 2013. p. 16–30. Tables 2A and 2B.

susceptible breakpoints for other diseases from the Clinical and Laboratory Standards Institute (CLSI) VET01-A4 document.[25] While none of these antimicrobials have an approved CLSI breakpoint for treatment of any disease due to treponemes, it is at least possible to compare the minimal inhibitory concentration (MIC) values for 90% of the tested organisms (MIC_{90}) to established susceptible breakpoints for other veterinary diseases to rule out potential antimicrobials for which the MIC values are well out of the range of potential therapeutic effect. However, caution is appropriate because the disease is different, the pathogen is different (and therefore the drug pharmacodynamics may be substantially different), the site-specific pharmacokinetics may be different (both because of site and regimen), and there is a lack of correlation of MICs with the therapeutic regimen and clinical results. Also, in lacking CLSI-approved standards for this organism, the testing methods may give different results compared with those of other methods based on multiple criteria. Even between the 2 referenced papers, there are slight differences in the inocula and media. It cannot be overemphasized that although the investigators made significant efforts to provide appropriate susceptibility testing methods, these have not undergone the CLSI approval process.

Therefore, in evaluating **Table 2**, an MIC_{90} well above the range of the ones established for systemic therapy for other diseases would likely require the potential for significantly higher drug concentrations at the site of infection to suggest consideration of use (eg, topical application at high concentrations), and therefore suggest significantly lower optimism for potential efficacy after systemic administration. For a discussion on the application of susceptibility testing in bovine therapeutics, see the article by Lubbers elsewhere in this issue.

The MIC_{90} values for erythromycin, oxytetracycline, penicillin, spectinomycin, and gamithromycin (Zactran) are below the CLSI-susceptible breakpoints approved for these drugs in other diseases, in some cases in other animal species. Of these, oxytetracycline, penicillin, spectinomycin, and gamithromycin have breakpoints established for a specific regimen against bovine respiratory disease (BRD) based on systemic administration. Oxytetracycline and penicillin are CLSI generic BRD breakpoints based on pathogen MIC distributions along with pharmacokinetic and pharmacodynamic properties of the antimicrobials against bacterial pathogens, but without clinical trial correlation to clinical outcome. For all drugs with MIC_{90} values that suggest potential systemic efficacy, all but oxytetracycline have MIC_{90} values very close to the MBC_{90} values, suggesting bactericidal activity against the pathogen. Confirmation of bactericidal activity through kill curve assays would be helpful in this interpretation. For these drugs, the close proximity of the MIC_{90} values to the susceptible breakpoints for other bovine diseases suggests that evaluating systemic efficacy would be worthwhile; however, systemic efficacy is not assured.

Another issue in considering application of nonapproved breakpoints is topical versus systemic therapy; there are no CLSI veterinary breakpoints that are approved for topical therapy. For example, the comparison of lincomycin MIC values to the available veterinary clindamycin-susceptible breakpoint (clindamycin for canine skin and soft tissue disease) in **Table 2** would suggest a poor prognosis for efficacy after systemic therapy, yet there are 2 clinical trials reported in **Table 1** that show significant topical efficacy for lincomycin in PDD.

Recurrence of Papillomatous Digital Dermatitis

The treatment successes reported in the literature may not result in continued absence of disease. In a long-term monitoring study of 39 cases of PDD initially treated with topical lincomycin, Berry and colleagues[22] observed that 54% required re-treatment on at least 1 occasion during the 341-day monitoring period. An early report of the spread of PDD through California dairy herds reported a 48% recurrence and new lesion rate in cows initially responding to injectable penicillin G or ceftiofur, topical formaldehyde or hydrochloric acid, or surgical excision.[4] These treatments are not included in the evidence table because of lack of information about the studies. One other reference to systemic ceftiofur efficacy for PDD was found in the lay literature, but communication with the investigator confirmed that although randomized with negative controls, the subjective evaluators were not masked.[26]

Potential for Milk Residues from Topical Papillomatous Digital Dermatitis Therapy

As PDD occurs in both lactating and dry dairy cows, the potential for milk residues resulting from topical treatment is a concern. This potential was investigated by Britt and colleagues[27] related to oxytetracycline in milk after 2 topical treatments for PDD. Analysis was by high-performance liquid chromatography (HPLC) (limit of detection of 3.3 ppb) and a tetracycline screening test (90% sensitivity at $\geq$19 ppb), both performed at the US Food and Drug Administration' (FDA's) Center for Veterinary Medicine. The tolerance for residues consisting of the sum of residues of the tetracyclines in milk is 300 ppb.[28]

Treatment 1 (N = 16) consisted of approximately 15 mL of an oxytetracycline solution, 100 mg/mL, applied topically with a garden sprayer twice daily for 7 days. Samples were obtained 24, 48, 72, 96, and 120 hours after the first spray application. Of the 80 samples collected for this treatment, 72 had no oxytetracycline detected and 8 had residues detectable by HPLC at concentrations from less than 1 to 6.7 ppb. The screening test gave negative results for all 80 samples.

Treatment 2 (N = 12) consisted of 20 mL of an oxytetracycline solution, 100 mg/mL, soaked in cotton, applied to the lesion and held on by tape until the tape deteriorated and fell off. The PDD lesions were sprayed immediately after milking. Samples were obtained 17, 48, 72, and 120 hours after bandage application. Of the 48 samples for treatment 2, no oxytetracycline was detected in 39 samples by HPLC, and concentrations ranging from 3.5 to 12 ppb were detected in the other 9 samples. All 48 samples gave negative result by the screening test.

These results suggest that the chance for a violative residue in the bulk tank is minimal with the stated uses of oxytetracycline for the treatment of PDD. However, the use will result in oxytetracycline being used in the parlor, so contamination of milking equipment, and therefore potentially the milk, must be avoided. Also, the variation encountered in the trial does not preclude that a small proportion of the population may display residues in milk that would exceed the acceptable tolerance. This study related to oxytetracycline should not be extrapolated to indicate that other topical treatments would have similar residue characteristics. This is especially true for treatments such as lincomycin, where the lack of a lactating dairy cattle label for any purpose results in an effective tolerance of zero (any detected). With today's testing technology, such as mass spectrometry, the potential for residue detection cannot be dismissed.

Effect of Site of Infection

Hernandez and Shearer[29] evaluated the effect of topical treatment of PDD with topical application of an oxytetracycline solution, 25 mg/mL, based on the location of the lesion. Cows with PDD lesions on one hindfoot, characterized as early or mature according to study criteria and with lesion size determined, were classified as the lesion being located on the interdigital cleft (n = 14), heels,[30] or dewclaw.[26] Treatment of all lesions consisted of daily topical application of the oxytetracycline solution by sprayer, after cleaning with water, for 5 days. Treatment was stopped for 2 days, then resumed for an additional 3 days. The proportion of cows with mature lesions or with large lesion sizes were not different between groups at the time of treatment initiation. Lesions were examined at 14 and 30 days after initiation of treatment. Evaluation of both pain scores and lesion size indicated that cows with lesions on the interdigital cleft were less likely to respond to treatment when compared with cows with lesions on the heels or dewclaw. On days 14 and 30, the proportion of cows with pain scores greater than 0 for lesions located in the interdigital cleft (85% and 91%, respectively) were greater than for cows with lesions located on the dewclaw (18% and 24%, respectively), at $P<.05$.

Consideration of Human Treponema Infections

Parallels in the treatment of treponeme-associated diseases in humans may be of interest in evaluating potential systemic therapies for PDD. *Treponema pallidum* is the causative agent of syphilis, for which penicillin G has long been the mainstay of treatment. With issues of treatment due to penicillin G allergies, the antimicrobials tetracycline, doxycycline, erythromycin, azithromycin, and ceftriaxone have been evaluated and used for therapy.[30] However, macrolide resistance was reported in Irish and US isolates of *T pallidum* in 2004 and linked to a mutation in the 23S ribosomal RNA genes.[31] This resistance is now appearing in multiple locations around the world. Yaws, bejel (endemic syphilis), and pinta are the other three classic human treponematoses.[32] All human treponematoses share the characteristic of manifestation of multiple stages involving the skin. Single-dose azithromycin is being considered a pivotal tool to achieve worldwide eradication of yaws by 2020.

The parallels between PDD and human treponematoses are striking, as are the antimicrobials considered vital in treating the primary pathogen. The development of widespread resistance to macrolides in human therapy for *T pallidum* perhaps underscores a warning to wisely approach control measures. The single-injection macrolides currently available for respiratory disease therapy in cattle present challenges in both slaughter and milk withdrawal times in lactating dairy cattle, but may hold promise for limited individual animal therapy in beef cattle outbreaks, such as in feedlots.

INFECTIOUS PODODERMATITIS (FOOT ROT, ACUTE INTERDIGITAL NECROBACILLOSIS)

IP, when compared with PDD, has the advantage of multiple labels approved for therapy for this disease in cattle. For some of these drugs, there is the ready availability of freedom of information (FOI) summaries detailing pivotal studies demonstrating substantial evidence of efficacy.

Randomized, Masked, Prospective Trials with Negative Controls for Systemic Therapy for Infectious Pododermatitis

In 1995, ceftiofur sodium (Naxcel) was granted a supplemental approval for the treatment of acute bovine interdigital necrobacillosis (foot rot, pododermatitis) associated with *Fusobacterium necrophorum* and *Bacteroides melaninogenicus*.[33] An induced model dose-finding study initially confirmed that both 1.1 and 2.2 mg/kg administered intramuscularly (IM) at 24-hour intervals for 3 days were equally effective in the treatment of IP. A multilocation dose confirmation study using the 1.1 mg/kg regimen was then conducted in 88 beef feedlot cattle and lactating dairy cows at 16 sites. As shown in **Table 3**, treatment with ceftiofur sodium was statistically significant in superiority to the negative control. Treatment success was based on a combination of a reduction in lameness score by 2 points with nil to moderate swelling and healed or healing lesions.

Table 3
Evidence from randomized, masked, prospective clinical trials for individual animal therapy of bovine infectious pododermatitis expressed as percentage success and NNT

Reference	Case Definition	Success Definition	N	Treatments	% with Positive Case Outcome	NNT
Ceftiofur sodium FOI (1995) Study 2	Lesions and lameness	Lesion, lameness, and swelling scores on day 7	45	Control: sterile water every 24 h for 3 d	14.0%	—
			43	1.1 mg/kg IM every 24 h	62.2%	2.07 (2)
CCFA FOI (2008)	Lameness, lesion, and swelling score of 2 or 3 in 1 foot only for 2 consecutive days	Reduction of 2 or more score for lameness; and swelling and lesion score 0 or 1 on day 7 in qualifying foot	89	Vehicle-treated control	13.2%	—
			88	CCFA-SS 6.6 mg CE/kg BW SC (base of ear) single injection day 0	58.4%	2.21 (2)
Florfenicol FOI (1999)	2 consecutive days of nonresolving lesions and lameness scores of 2 or greater	Day 0 lesion score $\geq$2 decreasing to 0 or 1; with reduction in lameness score of 2 points or returning to 0	90	Control: same volume and timing as for the florfenicol IM regimen	0.0%	—
				Florfenicol 20 mg/kg IM dosed twice in a 48-h interval	77.0%	1.30 (1)
				Florfenicol 40 mg/kg SC single dose	77.0%	1.30 (1)
Tulathromycin FOI (2008) Study 1	Lameness, lesion, and swelling score of 2 or 3 in 1 foot only for 2 consecutive days	Reduction from day 0–7 of 2 or more scores in lameness, and swelling & lesion scores of 0 or 1 on day 7 in the qualifying foot	50	Control: saline SC single injection on day 0	8.0%	—
			50	Tulathromycin (2.5 mg/kg) SC single injection on day 0	60.0%	1.93 (2)
Tulathromycin FOI (2008) Study 2	Lameness, lesion, and swelling score of 2 or 3 in 1 foot only for 2 consecutive days	Reduction from day 0–7 of 2 or more scores in lameness, and swelling & lesion scores of 0 or 1 on day 7 in the qualifying foot	34	Control: saline SC single injection on day 0	50.0%	—
			36	Tulathromycin (2.5 mg/kg) SC single injection on day 0	83.3%	3.00 (3)
Morck and colleagues,[42] 1998	Acute necrosis of skin causing swelling and lameness for a duration of 3 or more days	Lameness score 0 on day 4 and not re-treated for interdigital phlegmon within 10 d of initial treatment	50	Ceftiofur (1.0 mg/kg of BW IM every 24 h for 3 d	73.0%	—
			50	Oxytetracycline (6.6 mg/kg) IM every 24 h for 3 d	68.0%	—

Abbreviations: BW, body weight; CCFA, ceftiofur crystalline free acid; SC, subcutaneous.
Data from Refs. [33,35,37,38]

Ceftiofur hydrochloride (Excenel sterile suspension) received supplemental approval for cattle in 1998. It carries the same label indication for IP as does ceftiofur sodium based on therapeutic equivalence through pharmacokinetic studies.[34] A new formulation of ceftiofur hydrochloride was approved in 2008 (Excenel RTU EZ), which was confirmed as effective for all label indications for the previous formulation through a plasma bioequivalence approach.[35]

In 2008, another formulation of ceftiofur, ceftiofur crystalline free acid (CCFA, Excede), received supplemental approval for the treatment of bovine foot rot (interdigital necrobacillosis) associated with *F necrophorum* and *Porphyromonas levii* in beef, nonlactating dairy, and lactating dairy cattle.[36] The dose confirmation study involved 177 cattle, which included 70 beef steers and heifers and 107 lactating dairy cattle. Study entry was based on the requirement for an elevated lameness score, swelling score, and lesion score for 2 consecutive days. Success on day 7 of the study required a greater than or equal to 2 score reduction in lameness (0 to 3 scale with 0 being normal), plus swelling and lesion scores of 0 or 1, on 0 to 3 and 0 to 4 scales, respectively. The treated animals had statistically significant improvements in clinical success rates, as reported in **Table 3**.

Florfenicol (Nuflor) is labeled for the treatment of bovine interdigital phlegmon (foot rot, acute interdigital necrobacillosis, IP) associated with *F necrophorum* and *B melaninogenicus*. The clinical study contained in the 1999 supplemental approval FOI summary involved 90 crossbred beef steers with a mean weight of 436 kg.[37] As reported in **Table 3**, the study involved a saline control group and a group for each of the two florfenicol label regimens. To be enrolled, the cattle had to display 2 days of nonresolving lesions and lameness based on the study scoring criteria of 0–4 for lesions and 0 to 3 for lameness, with 0 being normal for both scales. To be classified as a success on day 7, the lesion score must have decreased from ≥ 2 on day zero to a score of 0 or 1, and the lameness scores must have decreased by at least 2 points. On day 7, 77% of the study animals in both florfenicol treatment groups met success criteria, while none of the negative controls were successes. There was no statistical difference between florfenicol treatment groups, but both were statistically significantly different from the control group.

The 2008 supplemental approval of tulathromycin (Draxxin) for the treatment of bovine foot rot (interdigital necrobacillosis) associated with *F necrophorum* and *P levii* in beef and nonlactating dairy cattle reports the results of 2 studies.[38] Each study is identically structured, with cattle entering the study based on lameness, swelling, and lesion scores for 1 foot. Once entered into the study on study day 0, the criteria for treatment success were applied on day 7. A treatment success required at least a 2 score reduction on a 0 to 3 lameness score scale where 0 indicated no lameness noted and 3 meant holding up the foot with reluctance to put weight on the foot or move. A success was also required to have a swelling score of 0, indicating no swelling, and a lesion score of 0, indicating no lesion. The differences between saline control cattle and cattle treated with tulathromycin, as reported in **Table 3**, were statistically significant in both studies.

Other antimicrobials also have labels for the treatment of IP as found on the "Animal Drugs @ FDA" site, which is an online searchable version of the FDA "*Green Book*" containing veterinary labels.[39] These labels include oxytetracycline, tylosin, sulfadimethoxine, sulfabromomethazine, sulfaethoxypyridazine, and sulfamethazine. The best search term for this site is "foot rot," although results are also delivered for "foot-rot" and "pododermatitis." The presence of a label in this database does not indicate that the label is currently marketed, only that it is approved and has not been withdrawn by the company; some labels are present on the site with an indication that the label has been withdrawn by the company. Most of these labels are of a sufficient age such that the original freedom of information (FOI) summary is not available electronically on the FDA FOI site.[40] In addition, other antimicrobials without approved labels specifically for IP have been used for therapy, including formulations of penicillin G. According to the Animal Medicinal Drug Use Clarification Act regulations, the veterinarian must first consider if labeled products are effective when used according to label.[41]

In contrast to the pivotal clinical trials available for ceftiofur, florfenicol, and tulathromycin, clinical data to support the common use of other labeled antimicrobials for the treatment of IP are much less robust. At present, there are 50, 100, 200, and 300 mg/mL oxytetracycline products that are labeled for "treatment of … foot-rot and diphtheria caused by *Fusobacterium necrophorum*…" There is a published comparative trial of oxytetracycline and ceftiofur sodium that meets the reporting criteria for this review, although without a negative control.[42] Morck and colleagues[42] compared ceftiofur sodium, 1.0 mg/kg IM every 24 hours for 3 days, to oxytetracycline, 6.6 mg/kg IM every 24 hours for 3 days. This oxytetracycline regimen does not meet the current recommended uses of oxytetracycline as defined by route or dose. However, based on lameness scores and lack of re-treatment within 10 days of initial treatment, these ceftiofur sodium and oxytetracycline regimens were not statistically different in feedlot cattle, at 73.0% and 68% success, respectively. While not a clinical trial powered as to assure demonstration of non-inferiority of either product, these results do suggest that oxytetracycline is effective in the treatment of IP based on very similar results to ceftiofur, which has demonstrated efficacy in multiple trials utilizing different formulations.

In vitro Susceptibility Testing of F Necrophorum

While susceptibility testing data for bovine IP isolates of *F necrophorum* are lacking, there are data related to other bovine isolates of this pathogen. Mateos and colleagues[43] tested multiple antimicrobial agents against *F necrophorum* isolates from liver abscesses in cattle. As summarized in **Table 4**, ampicillin, oxytetracycline,

Table 4
MIC$_{50}$ and MIC$_{90}$ for *F necrophorum* isolates as related to CLSI veterinary breakpoints for other diseases expressed as MIC

	MIC$_{50}$ and MIC$_{90}$ Values for *Fusobacterium* Isolates		
Drug	MIC$_{50}$ (μg/mL)	MIC$_{90}$ (μg/mL)	CLSI Veterinary Breakpoints for Other Diseases (μg/mL)
Ampicillin	0.01	0.06	0.25[a]
Chlortetracycline	0.125	1	4[b]
Gentamicin	16	64	2[c]
Oxytetracycline	0.5	2	2[d]
Penicillin G	0.01	0.01	0.25[d]
Sulfadimethoxine	16	32	256[e]
Tylosin	0.5	1	___

[a] CLSI susceptible breakpoint for canine skin and soft tissue and equine respiratory disease. The swine respiratory disease breakpoint is 0.5.
[b] CLSI breakpoint for chlortetracycline is adapted from the human tetracycline breakpoint and has not been assigned a veterinary generic breakpoint as has been done for oxytetracycline.
[c] CLSI susceptible breakpoint for specific organisms in canine and equine systemic disease.
[d] CLSI susceptible breakpoint for bovine respiratory disease.
[e] CLSI human derived breakpoint for sulfasoxizole as the representative for nonpotentiated sulfas. This breakpoint has not been correlated with any veterinary clinical outcomes.

penicillin G, and sulfadimethoxine seem to have MIC_{90} values which appear favorable in relation to CLSI susceptibility breakpoints derived for other infections. Chlortetracycline seems to be favorable in relation to the human-adapted CLSI breakpoint, but that breakpoint comes from systemic human therapy and chlortetracycline is administered orally in cattle with poor bioavailability. In contrast, the oxytetracycline CLSI-approved breakpoint for BRD is based on bovine pharmacokinetics and the pharmacodynamics of oxytetracycline against bacterial pathogens. This origin of the oxytetracycline breakpoint gives more comfort to extrapolation of the BRD breakpoint to other diseases, such as IP. These susceptibility data support common approaches to treating IP with a sulfa formulation, oxytetracycline, or a formulation of penicillin G. However, readily available clinical confirmation of efficacy is only available for ceftiofur, tulathromycin, and florfenicol. Clinical trial confirmation for healing or prevention of IP cases while cattle are being administered oxytetracycline or chlortetracycline in the feed were not detected in the literature search for this article.

SUMMARY

Clinical evidence presented here was limited to randomized, prospective clinical trials conducted in naturally occurring disease with negative controls and masked subjective evaluators. In the case of PDD, these trials support the use of topical tetracycline and oxytetracycline, lincomycin, a copper-containing preparation, and a nonantimicrobial cream. Susceptibility testing of *Treponema* spp isolates and parallels with *Treponema*-associated disease in humans supports the potential for systemic use of macrolides and some β-lactams, but clinical trial confirmation would be appropriate. The therapy for PDD is complicated by a multipathogen cause, and recurrence of disease after an initial clinical resolution is a common problem. There were no clinical data found meeting criteria for inclusion in this article which support the systemic therapy of PDD. However, susceptibility testing and consideration of human treponematoses therapy suggest that clinical evaluation of drugs such as ceftiofur and macrolides should be furthered.

In the case of individual therapy for IP, trial evidence is available to support systemic treatment with ceftiofur, florfenicol, tulathromycin, and oxytetracycline. Clinical trial evidence was not readily available for IP standards such as penicillin G, sulfadimethoxine, and tylosin, although consideration of susceptibility testing, with the many appropriate caveats, seems to support the clinical impressions that lead to their common use for therapy for IP.

REFERENCES

1. Sargeant JM, O'Connor AM, Gardner IA, et al. The REFLECT statement: reporting guidelines for randomized controlled trials in livestock and food safety: explanation and elaboration. J Food Prot 2010;73(3):579–603.
2. Cook RJ, Sackett DL. The number needed to treat: a clinically useful measure of treatment effect. BMJ 1995;310(6977):452–4.
3. Blowey RW, Sharp MW. Digital dermatitis in dairy cattle. Vet Rec 1988;122(21): 505–8.
4. Read DH, Walker RL. Papillomatous digital dermatitis (footwarts) in California dairy cattle: clinical and gross pathologic findings. J Vet Diagn Invest 1998;10(1):67–76.
5. Blowey RW, Sharp MW, Done SH. Digital dermatitis. Vet Rec 1992;131(2):39.
6. Blowey RW, Done SH, Cooley W. Observations on the pathogenesis of digital dermatitis in cattle. Vet Rec 1994;135(5):115–7.

7. Dhawi A, Hart CA, Demirkan I, et al. Bovine digital dermatitis and severe virulent ovine foot rot: a common spirochaetal pathogenesis. Vet J 2005;169(2):232–41.
8. Logue DN, Offer JE, Laven RA, et al. Digital dermatitis–the aetiological soup. Vet J 2005;170(1):12–3.
9. Holzhauer M, Bartels CJ, Bergsten C, et al. The effect of an acidified, ionized copper sulphate solution on digital dermatitis in dairy cows. Vet J 2012;193(3): 659–63.
10. Holzhauer M, Dopfer D, de Boer J, et al. Effects of different intervention strategies on the incidence of papillomatous digital dermatitis in dairy cows. Vet Rec 2008; 162(2):41–6.
11. Dopfer D, Holzhauer M, Boven M. The dynamics of digital dermatitis in populations of dairy cattle: model-based estimates of transition rates and implications for control. Vet J 2012;193(3):648–53.
12. Hoffman A. Footbaths for the treatment or control of hairy heel warts (digital dermatitis) in dairy herds: summary of seven studies. Pullman(Washington): Washington State University Veterinary Medicine Extension Ag Animal Health Spotlight; 2012. p. 6.
13. Laven RA, Logue DN. Treatment strategies for digital dermatitis for the UK. Vet J 2006;171(1):79–88.
14. Logue DN, Gibert T, Parkin T, et al. A field evaluation of a footbathing solution for the control of digital dermatitis in cattle. Vet J 2012;193(3):664–8.
15. Speijers MH, Baird LG, Finney GA, et al. Effectiveness of different footbath solutions in the treatment of digital dermatitis in dairy cows. J Dairy Sci 2010;93(12): 5782–91.
16. Speijers MH, Finney GA, McBride J, et al. Effectiveness of different footbathing frequencies using copper sulfate in the control of digital dermatitis in dairy cows. J Dairy Sci 2012;95(6):2955–64.
17. Cook NB, Rieman J, Gomez A, et al. Observations on the design and use of footbaths for the control of infectious hoof disease in dairy cattle. Vet J 2012;193(3):669–73.
18. Cutler JH, Cramer G, Walter JJ, et al. Randomized clinical trial of tetracycline hydrochloride bandage and paste treatments for resolution of lesions and pain associated with digital dermatitis in dairy cattle. J Dairy Sci 2013;96(12):7550–7.
19. Moore DA, Berry SL, Truscott ML, et al. Efficacy of a nonantimicrobial cream administered topically for treatment of digital dermatitis in dairy cattle. J Am Vet Med Assoc 2001;219(10):1435–8.
20. Hernandez J, Shearer JK, Elliott JB. Comparison of topical application of oxytetracycline and four nonantibiotic solutions for treatment of papillomatous digital dermatitis in dairy cows. J Am Vet Med Assoc 1999;214(5):688–90.
21. Berry SL, Read DH, Walker RL, et al. Clinical, histologic, and bacteriologic findings in dairy cows with digital dermatitis (footwarts) one month after topical treatment with lincomycin hydrochloride or oxytetracycline hydrochloride. J Am Vet Med Assoc 2010;237(5):555–60.
22. Berry SL, Read DH, Famula TR, et al. Long-term observations on the dynamics of bovine digital dermatitis lesions on a California dairy after topical treatment with lincomycin HCl. Vet J 2012;193(3):654–8.
23. Evans NJ, Brown JM, Demirkan I, et al. In vitro susceptibility of bovine digital dermatitis associated spirochaetes to antimicrobial agents. Vet Microbiol 2009; 136(1–2):115–20.
24. Evans NJ, Brown JM, Hartley C, et al. Antimicrobial susceptibility testing of bovine digital dermatitis treponemes identifies macrolides for in vivo efficacy testing. Vet Microbiol 2012;160(3–4):496–500.

25. CLSI. VET01–A4 performance standards for antimicrobial disk and dilution susceptibility tests for bacteria isolated from animals; approved standard – fourth edition. Wayne (PA): Clinical and Laboratory Standards Institute; 2013.

26. Guterbock W, Borelli C. Footwart trial report. Western Dairyman 1995;17.

27. Britt JS, Carson MC, von Bredow JD, et al. Antibiotic residues in milk samples obtained from cows after treatment for papillomatous digital dermatitis. J Am Vet Med Assoc 1999;215(6):833–6.

28. FDA/CVM. Title 21-food and drugs, Chapter 1-Food and Drug Administration Department of Health and Human Services, subchapter E - animal drugs, feeds, and related products, part 556-tolerances for residues of new animal drugs, subpart B - specific tolerances for residues of new animal drugs. Accessed January 2, 2015. Available at: http://www.accessdata.fda.gov/scripts/cdrh/cfdocs/cfcfr/CFRSearch.cfm?CFRPart=556.

29. Hernandez J, Shearer JK. Efficacy of oxytetracycline for treatment of papillomatous digital dermatitis lesions on various anatomic locations in dairy cows. J Am Vet Med Assoc 2000;216(8):1288–90.

30. Holman KM, Hook EW 3rd. Clinical management of early syphilis. Expert Rev Anti Infect Ther 2013;11(8):839–43.

31. Lukehart SA, Godornes C, Molini BJ, et al. Macrolide resistance in *Treponema pallidum* in the United States and Ireland. N Engl J Med 2004;351(2):154–8.

32. Giacani L, Lukehart SA. The endemic treponematoses. Clin Microbiol Rev 2014;27(1):89–115.

33. FDA/CVM. Supplemental New Animal Drug Application, NADA 140-338, Naxcel sterile powder, for the treatment of interdigital necrobacillosis (foot rot, pododermatitis). CVM FOI. 1995. Accessed January 2, 2015. Available at: http://www.fda.gov/AnimalVeterinary/Products/ApprovedAnimalDrugProducts/FOIADrugSummaries/ucm049774.htm.

34. FDA/CVM. Supplement to NADA 140-890, Excenel sterile suspension (ceftiofur hydrochloride injection) "For the treatment of bovine respiratory disease (BRD) associated with *Pasteurella multocida*, *P. haemolytica*, and *Haemophilus somnus* and for the treatment of acute bovine interdigital necrobacillosis (foot rot) associated with *Fusobacterium necrophorum* and *Bacteroides melaninogenicus*." 1998. Accessed January 2, 2015. Available at: http://www.fda.gov/downloads/AnimalVeterinary/Products/ApprovedAnimalDrugProducts/FOIADrugSummaries/ucm059122.pdf.

35. FDA/CVM. Original new animal drug application 141-288 Excenel RTU EZ sterile suspension for injection swine and cattle (beef, non-lactating dairy, and lactating dairy). 2008. Accessed January 2, 2015. Available at: http://www.fda.gov/downloads/AnimalVeterinary/Products/ApprovedAnimalDrugProducts/FOIADrugSummaries/UCM208544.pdf.

36. FDA/CVM. Supplemental New Animal Drug Application, NADA 141-209, Excede sterile suspension, for the treatment of bovine foot rot (interdigital necrobacillosis). CVM FOI. 2008. Accessed August 14, 2014. Available at: http://www.fda.gov/downloads/AnimalVeterinary/Products/ApprovedAnimalDrugProducts/FOIADrugSummaries/ucm117772.pdf.

37. FDA/CVM. Supplemental New Animal Drug Application, NADA 141-063, Nuflor injectable solution, for the trea5tment of bovine interdigital phlegmon (foot rot, acute interdigital necrobacillosis, infectious pododermatitis). CVM FOI. 1999. Accessed January 2, 2015. Available at: http://www.fda.gov/downloads/AnimalVeterinary/Products/ApprovedAnimalDrugProducts/FOIADrugSummaries/ucm116742.pdf.

38. FDA/CVM. Supplemental New Animal Drug Application, NADA 141–244, Draxxin injectable solution, for the treatment of bovine foot rot (interdigital necrobacillosis). CVM FOI. 2008. Accessed January 2, 2015. Available at: http://www.fda.gov/AnimalVeterinary/Products/ApprovedAnimalDrugProducts/FOIADrugSummaries/ucm080277.htm.

39. FDA/CVM. Food and Drug Administration Center for Veterinary Medicine, Animal Drugs @ FDA. 2014. Accessed January 2, 2015. Available at: http://www.accessdata.fda.gov/scripts/animaldrugsatfda/.

40. FDA/CVM. Food and Drug Administration Center for Veterinary Medicine FOIA Drug Summaries. 2014. Accessed January 2, 2015. Available at: http://www.fda.gov/AnimalVeterinary/Products/ApprovedAnimalDrugProducts/FOIADrugSummaries/default.htm.

41. FDA/CVM. Food and Drug Administration Center for Veterinary Medicine final rule - extralabel drug use in animals. Washington DC: Federal Register; 1996. p. 57731–46.

42. Morck DW, Olson ME, Louie TJ, et al. Comparison of ceftiofur sodium and oxytetracycline for treatment of acute interdigital phlegmon (foot rot) in feedlot cattle. J Am Vet Med Assoc 1998;212(2):254–7.

43. Mateos E, Piriz S, Valle J, et al. Minimum inhibitory concentrations for selected antimicrobial agents against *Fusobacterium necrophorum* isolated from hepatic abscesses in cattle and sheep. J Vet Pharmacol Ther 1997;20(1):21–3.

A Review of the Expected Effects of Antimicrobials in Bovine Respiratory Disease Treatment and Control Using Outcomes from Published Randomized Clinical Trials with Negative Controls

Keith D. DeDonder, MS, DVM*, Michael D. Apley, DVM, PhD

KEYWORDS

- Antimicrobial drugs • Antibiotic susceptibility • Antibiotic resistance
- Bovine respiratory disease • Number needed to treat • Randomized clinical trial
- Evidence based medicine

KEY POINTS

- The randomized clinical trial (RCT) is the gold standard for efficacy determination.
- RCTs with negative (no treatment) controls are not clouded by a control group treatment effect.
- Absolute risk reduction (ARR) is the difference in the probabilities of an event in the control and treatment groups and is estimated as the corresponding difference in the event rates.
- Number needed to treat (NNT) is the reciprocal of the ARR.
- NNT is more clinically intuitive because it describes the effect in terms of the number of patients a clinician needs to treat to expect a given (typically positive) outcome.

INTRODUCTION

Bovine respiratory disease (BRD) is a multifactorial disease that has been well described by many researchers as a complex or syndrome involving an interaction of stressors, viruses, and bacteria. Despite decades of dedicated research, BRD

ICCM, Kansas State University College of Veterinary Medicine, P200 Mosier Hall, Manhattan, KS 66506, USA
* Corresponding author.
E-mail address: kdd5257@vet.k-state.edu

Vet Clin Food Anim 31 (2015) 97–111
http://dx.doi.org/10.1016/j.cvfa.2014.11.003
0749-0720/15/$ – see front matter © 2015 Elsevier Inc. All rights reserved.

remains a major disease in all types of beef and dairy production systems, with an estimated global economic impact in excess of $3 billion per year.[1] Antimicrobial administration is a mainstay in both the control of disease in populations at high risk of BRD and in the therapeutic treatment of acute clinical disease. The pipeline of novel antimicrobial classes for therapy for BRD has remained dry, however, since the introduction of enrofloxacin (Baytril 100, Bayer Animal Health, Shawnee Mission, Kansas) in 1998. Therefore, the judicious use of antimicrobials in both human and animal health remains paramount to ensure efficacy of treatment remains acceptable.

The objective of this article is to evaluate the use of antimicrobials for therapy for BRD through the lens of a cumulative review of published RCTs investigating the effects of an antimicrobial drug for treatment or control of BRD against a negative control. The NNT is used to describe these trials.[2] There are many ways to express the value of an active treatment over that of its control group, such as odds ratios and risk reduction. NNT is the reciprocal of the ARR, which is the difference in the probabilities of an event in the control and treatment groups and is estimated as the corresponding difference in these event rates. The NNT statistic has the major advantage of being more straightforward to readers less versed in thinking of events (clinical outcome) in terms of probabilities. NNT is more easily interpreted by practicing clinicians and speaks in terms of number of treatments needed to make a difference in 1 patient. The use of NNT, by expressing the effect of the drug in relation to disease recovery of negative controls over the same period, also incorporates the severity of the disease challenge into the estimate of drug effect. Therefore, the use of the NNT value must be carefully relegated to the disease, regimen, animal species, and specific disease challenge.

ANCILLARY THERAPY USE IN BOVINE RESPIRATORY DISEASE

A systematic review was conducted and published in 2012 by Francoz and colleagues[3] on the use of ancillary drugs in the treatment of BRD. Although finding few reliable and consistent data, they concluded that there were not enough data at that time to recommend the use of any ancillary therapy alongside antimicrobials in the treatment of BRD. Using the same search criteria as performed in that study, the authors were unable to identify any recent publications of relevance to expand that conversation; therefore, interested readers should consult that publication. Likewise, no clinical trial data addressing the use of more than 1 antimicrobial at a time versus a single antimicrobial for therapy for BRD were found. The focus of this review is, therefore, limited to the use of antimicrobials alone in the treatment of BRD.

ANTIMICROBIAL USE IN BOVINE RESPIRATORY DISEASE

The prospective, masked, RCT conducted in naturally occurring disease is the gold standard for the evaluation of efficacy for disease intervention in both human and veterinary medical clinical research. In regard to naturally occurring BRD studies of antimicrobial efficacy, the literature is divided into those using a negative control and those comparing the test article to a positive control. When using a positive control treatment, the goal of the experiment is to prove either superiority or noninferiority, either of which requires different study designs. The lack of a significant difference in treatment outcomes in a trial, which was not adequately designed to demonstrate noninferiority, cannot necessarily be interpreted as equivalence of the treatments. Analysis and interpretation of trials with positive controls provide many challenges and are beyond the scope of this article. An excellent meta-analysis was recently performed in this area and readers wishing for that scope should refer to the article by

O'Connor and colleagues.[4] Briefly, they used a mixed treatment comparison meta-analysis to compare the efficacy of antimicrobial treatments of BRD.[5] In addition to including trials using a negative control, their inclusion criteria and methods of analysis allowed the inclusion of study designs using a positive control as a treatment arm in their analysis. As such, the number of article inclusions was much larger than those included in this report. In **Fig. 1**, a visual network of the treatment arms compared in their meta-analysis is appreciated. Their publication offered comparisons of 60 trials of active drug to negative controls (including Freedom of Informations [FOI summaries]) and 33 comparisons of active-to-active (1 antimicrobial to another) controls. By means of their meta-analysis method, they were able to rank antimicrobial treatments of BRD by efficacy (**Fig. 2**). Using their rankings, with the published data available in the literature, tulathromycin ranks as the most efficacious treatment of BRD, and the older molecules, such as the ceftiofur formulations, trimethoprim and oxytetracycline, are among the least efficacious antimicrobial treatments of BRD. As pointed out by O'Connor and colleagues, a limitation not unique to their meta-analysis is that the analysis is limited to those data publically available. If more privately held trial data were offered, better estimates might be possible.

This article has not attempted to include those publications with a positive control because the authors are not attempting to compare efficacy between treatments, instead elucidating the actual effect gained from the use of an antimicrobial in therapy for or control of BRD. An alternate interpretation of results is possible when the control group is administered either no treatment or a sham, such as a saline injection, because comparisons to the control group are not clouded by an actual treatment effect. It is in this type of research where the true effect of the antimicrobial in that

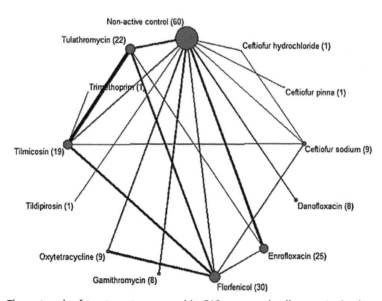

Fig. 1. The network of treatment arms used in O'Connor and colleagues' mixed treatment comparisons meta-analysis. The size of the dot is a relative indicator of the number of arms and the width of the lines is a relative indicator of the number of direct comparisons (number of arms). (*From* O'Connor AM, Coetzee JF, da Silva N, et al. A mixed treatment comparison meta-analysis of antibiotic treatments for bovine respiratory disease. Prev Vet Med 2013;110:80; with permission.)

Treatment		Ranking [95% Credibility Interval]
Tulathromycin	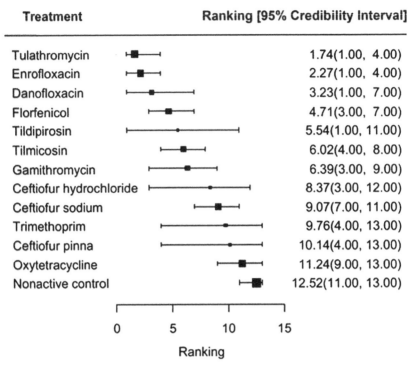	1.74(1.00, 4.00)
Enrofloxacin		2.27(1.00, 4.00)
Danofloxacin		3.23(1.00, 7.00)
Florfenicol		4.71(3.00, 7.00)
Tildipirosin		5.54(1.00, 11.00)
Tilmicosin		6.02(4.00, 8.00)
Gamithromycin		6.39(3.00, 9.00)
Ceftiofur hydrochloride		8.37(3.00, 12.00)
Ceftiofur sodium		9.07(7.00, 11.00)
Trimethoprim		9.76(4.00, 13.00)
Ceftiofur pinna		10.14(4.00, 13.00)
Oxytetracycline		11.24(9.00, 13.00)
Nonactive control		12.52(11.00, 13.00)

Ranking

Fig. 2. Ranking forest plot for treatment arms in O'Connor and colleagues' mixed treatment comparison meta-analysis of antibiotic protocols for BRD (mean rank and 95% credibility interval). (*From* O'Connor AM, Coetzee JF, da Silva N, et al. A mixed treatment comparison meta-analysis of antibiotic treatments for bovine respiratory disease. Prev Vet Med 2013;110:83; with permission from Elsevier.)

population of cattle is discerned. A certain level of spontaneous recovery is expected, due to misdiagnosis, a fully competent and successful immune response, or other factors that are unidentifiable. Therefore, comparing treated to untreated controls using the NNT allows an easily interpreted measurement of the antimicrobial effect in a specific clinical situation readily comprehended by veterinary practitioners and their clients alike.

DECIDING WHICH DATA DRIVE DECISIONS

A systematic review of the literature was performed using the online resources PubMed and Web of Knowledge in August of 2014, with similar search terms as outlined previously.[4] Studies were limited to those published in English and originating from North America. Criteria for inclusion in this review were that the publications must have been investigations into the treatment or control of BRD with an antimicrobial in a randomized, blinded, negative control field trial study design where subjective evaluators were masked and the disease was naturally occurring. Trials had to involve the administration of a single antimicrobial, with no ancillary therapy, either for treatment of naturally occurring BRD or in the control of naturally occurring BRD. Studies on the treatment of naturally occurring BRD must have involved animals that were not treated for control of BRD with an antimicrobial prior to or as part of the study. All trials involving positive controls or experimental challenge models were excluded. Additionally, publications were screened to ensure that they were not duplicative of FOI data, as was the case on many occasions.

Additionally, the FOI new animal drug application (NADA) summaries were searched on the Food and Drug Administration (FDA) Web site at the same time. Inclusions from the FOI summaries were efficacy trials (ETs), dose-response studies (DRSs), dose selection studies (DSSs), single-location field studies (FSs), and multilocation FSs (MLFSs). The only arms of dose selection studies reported are those that used current labeled dosages in the trial.

ARTICLE EXCLUSIONS

Articles from Hibbard and colleagues[6] and Hamm and colleagues,[7] which have been included in other review articles on antimicrobial treatment of BRD, were not included in this analysis because they were both found to be publications of data from their NADA FOI summaries. Additionally, in Hibbard and colleagues' article, the third trial was not included in the control analysis because the allocation to each treatment group was not presented. Percentages were given in tables of the trial outcome but did not allow the calculation of CIs. An article from Messersmith and colleagues[8] was not included because there was no mention of blinding the evaluators and in the article they actually mention tagging animals in accordance with their treatment, which suggests that evaluating investigators were aware of treatment during evaluation.

DATA EXTRACTION

Articles were organized by those investigations of BRD treatment efficacy or those reporting on efficacy of treatment for control of BRD. Outcome measures of treatment efficacy articles were treatment failures and mortality; those measurements in the control articles were morbidity. A summary of the individual animal treatment studies included in this report is in **Table 1**. All NADA approval studies are listed by the pharmaceutical company currently holding rights to the drug. The published journal articles are listed by the name of the company as it was when the study was supported and published. **Table 2** includes the publications providing data for the control/prevention portion of the analysis.

General information from FOI summaries and study reports was gathered, including authors, publication source, pharmaceutical sponsorship, treatment regimen, number of animals per treatment group, and treatment outcomes.

THE EFFECT OF ANTIMICROBIALS IN TREATING AND CONTROLLING BOVINE RESPIRATORY DISEASE

The box plots in **Figs. 3–5** represent a grouping of all the studies in regard to the trial outcomes of those animals receiving antimicrobials versus those receiving no treatment. A median spontaneous recovery rate of 24% was found across all trials in the control groups versus a 71% recovery rate of those treated with active ingredient for the therapeutic trials (see **Fig. 3**), indicating an increase of 47% recovery rate with the use of antimicrobials compared with a negative control. The median mortality rates by treatment group are 1% and 17% in treated and negative controls, respectively (see **Fig. 4**). The impact of treatment for control of BRD with an approved antimicrobial in cattle at high risk for developing disease is seen in **Fig. 5**. Treatment for

Table 1
Outline of publications presented for analysis in therapy for bovine respiratory disease in cattle from studies in North America

Drug	Date Approved or Published	Pharmaceutical Sponsor	Study Length (d)	Total Mortality (N)	Reported	Study Entry Criteria	Success Criteria
Ceftiofur sodium	1988	Zoetis	28	84	Yes	Rectal temp ≥104.5°F and 2 additional signs (depression, respiration, cough, anorexia)	Not stated
			28	88	Yes		
			28	88	Yes		
			28	88	Yes		
			28	88	Yes		
			28	405	Yes		
			28	405	Yes		
Florfenicol	Approved 1996	Merck	28	50	Yes	Acute clinical signs of pneumonia with rectal temp ≥104°F and respiratory rate ≥40 bpm	Not stated
Florfenicol	Approved 1996	Merck	15	95	Yes		
Florfenicol	Approved 1998	Merck	12	75	Yes		
Florfenicol	Approved 1998	Merck	12	75	Yes		
Florfenicol	Approved 1998	Merck	11	150	Yes		
Florfenicol	Approved 1998	Merck	11	150	Yes		
Ceftiofur CFA	Approved 2003	Zoetis	14	108	No	Rectal temp ≥104°F, respiratory index = 1, and depression index ≥1	Not a failure by day 14, and on day 14 had rectal temp <104°F; normal respiratory rates (respiratory index = 0); and no or mild depression (depression index ≤1)
Enrofloxacin	Approved 1996	Bayer	15	24	Yes	Rectal temp ≥104°F Clinical respiratory signs (increased rate and nasal discharge), poor attitude, and depression of appetite	Based on observations of attitude, appetite, rectal temp, and respiratory signs determined on day 6 and 28
Enrofloxacin	Approved 1998	Bayer	15	24	Yes		
Enrofloxacin	Approved 1996	Bayer	28	445	Yes		
Enrofloxacin	Approved 1998	Bayer	28	145	Yes		
Enrofloxacin	Approved 1996	Bayer	28	456	Yes		
Enrofloxacin	Approved 1998	Bayer	28	152	Yes		
Danofloxacin	Approved 2002	Zoetis	10	238	Yes	Rectal temp ≥104.5°F, increased rate and/or abnormal character of respiration, and depression	Response to therapy by 3–5 d without relapse by day 10 based on observation of respiratory signs, attitude, and rectal temp

Tulathromycin	Approved 2005	Zoetis	14	474	Yes	Attitude score ≥1, respiratory score = 1, and rectal temp ≥104°F	Survival through day 14 without being classified as a nonresponder (attitude score ≥1, respiration score = 1, and rectal temp of ≥104°F) or day 14 failure
Gamithromycin	Approved 2011	Merial	10	497	No	Exhibition of clinical signs of BRD (depression score ≥1, respiratory character score ≥1, and rectal temp ≥104°F)	Depression score = 0, respiratory character score = 0, and rectal temp <104°F
Gamithromycin	Approved 2012	Merial	10	242	No		
Gamithromycin	Approved 2012	Merial	10	260	No		
Tildipirosin	Approved 2012	Merck	14	600	Yes	Respiratory score ≥1, attitude score 2 or 3, and rectal temp ≥104°F	Respiratory score ≤1, attitude score of ≤1, and rectal temp <104°F
Danofloxacin	Approved 2011	Zoetis	10	240	No	Clinical signs of acute BRD (compromised respiration and depression) and rectal temp >104°F	Treatment success was based on respiratory signs, attitude, and rectal temp
Florfenicol	Approved 2008	Merck	11	244	No	Reference to previous FOI	Reference to previous FOI
Tulathromycin	Published 2005	Pfizer	14	480	Yes	Abnormal respiration (notable increase in rate and/or abnormal character of respiration); mild, moderate, or severe depression, and a rectal temp ≥104°F	Considered a success if not deemed a nonresponder (respiratory and attitude scores ≥1 and rectal temp ≥104°F) prior to day 14
Tilmicosin	Published 2005	Pfizer	14	480	Yes		
Florfenicol	Published 1997	Schering-Plough	45	125	Yes	Rectal temp ≥104.9°F for 2 consecutive days and an absence of abnormal clinical signs referable to organ systems other than the respiratory system	Absence of being classified a nonresponder (rectal temp ≥104°F and an absence of abnormal clinical signs referable to organ systems other than the respiratory system)

Abbreviations: bpm, breaths per minute; CFA, crystalline free acid; temp, temperature.

Pharmaceutical sponsors are listed by names as they exist today for each of the NADA studies. Where applicable, pharmaceutical companies are listed as they were named when sponsoring the independently published research studies.

Data from Refs.[12–24]

Table 2
Outline of publications presented for analysis in the control/prevention of bovine respiratory disease in cattle from studies in North America

Antimicrobial	Date	Pharma Sponsor	Study Length (d)	Total (N)	Case Definition
Ceftiofur CFA	Approved 2003	Zoetis	29	1504	Development of BRD (respiration score = 1, attitude score $\geq$1, and rectal temp $\geq$104°F) by day 14
Tulathromycin	Approved 2005	Zoetis	14	799	Attitude score $\geq$1, respiratory score = 1, and rectal temp $\geq$104°F
Florfenicol	Approved 1998	Merck	28	399	Clinical appearance, rectal temp,
Florfenicol	Approved 1998	Merck	28	198	respiratory rate, dyspnea, cough, and nasal discharge
Oxytetracycline	Approved 2003	Norbrook	30	1199	Clinical signs, such as poor general
Oxytetracycline	Approved 2003	Norbrook	30	1200	appearance, depressed attitude, and reluctance to move, and rectal temp $\geq$104°F
Tilmicosin	Approved 1996	Elanco	28	707	Clinical impression resulting from observing attitude, respiration rate, dyspnea, gauntness, and nasal and/or ocular discharge
Gamithromycin	Approved 2011	Merial	10	159	Mortality/euthanasia due to BRD
Gamithromycin	Approved 2011	Merial	10	308	or depression score $\geq$1 or respiratory score $\geq$2 and rectal temp $\geq$104°F
Tildipirosin	Approved 2012	Merck	14	773	Attitude score = 1 or 2 and rectal temp $\geq$104°F, or respiratory score = 2 and rectal temp $\geq$104°F, or respiratory score = 3 regardless of rectal temp, or attitude score of $\geq$3 regardless of rectal temp
Tulathromycin	Published 2005	Pfizer	14	819	Respiratory scores of 1 or attitude
Tilmicosin	Published 2005	Pfizer	14	817	scores of 1 and rectal temp $\geq$104°F
Tilmicosin	Published 1995	None	28	57	Clinical signs of BRD and a rectal
Tilmicosin	Published 1995	None	28	116	temp $\geq$103°F
Tilmicosin	Published 1995	None	56	121	
Tilmicosin	Published 1998	Elanco	28	1096	Variable at each site and treatment administration based on subjective assessment occurred
Ceftiofur CFA	Published 2008	Pfizer	69–83	1045	Clinical attitude score $\geq$1 and rectal temp $\geq$104°F
Oxytetracycline	Published 2013	Merck	24–49	3784	Rectal temp of $\geq$104°F and an absence of abnormal clinical signs directly attributable to organ systems other than the respiratory system

Pharmaceutical sponsors are listed by names as they exist today for each of the NADA studies. Where applicable, pharmaceutical companies are listed as they were named when sponsoring the independently published research studies.

Data from Refs.[5,14,15,18–20,25–30]

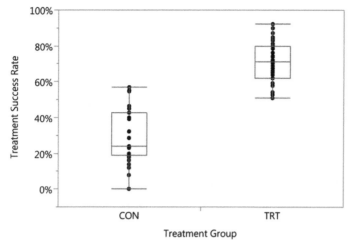

Fig. 3. Treatment success rate in all trials included in the therapeutic portion of the analysis. Control (CON) animals received either no treatment or sham-saline injection; treated (TRT) animals received an antimicrobial for the treatment of acute BRD.

control of BRD decreased the incidence of morbidity by more than half in these populations of cattle (22% in treated cattle vs 48% incidence in control cattle).

NUMBER NEEDED TO TREAT

Using the extracted data, a spreadsheet was constructed in Microsoft Excel (2013) with the information in **Tables 1** and **2** along with the outcomes of each individual trial. ARR, NNT, and their respective 95% CIs were calculated with the use of a spreadsheet calculator developed using the Newcombe-Wilson method without

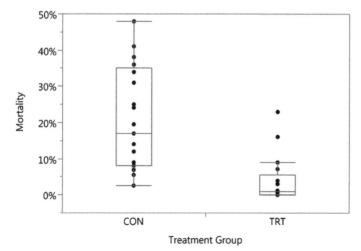

Fig. 4. Mortality incidence rates in all trials included in the therapeutic portion of the analysis. Control (CON) animals received either no treatment or sham-saline injection; treated (TRT) animals received an antimicrobial for the treatment of acute BRD.

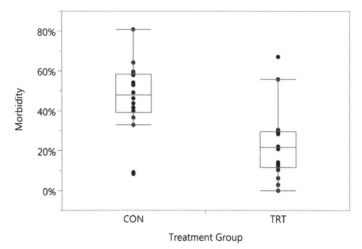

Fig. 5. Morbidity incidence rates in all trials included in the mass medication portion of the analysis. Control (CON) animals received either no treatment or sham-saline injection; treated (TRT) animals received an antimicrobial for the prevention/control of BRD.

continuity correction.[9] The outputted ARR and CIs were inputted into JMP 11.0.0 (SAS Institute, Cary, North Carolina) for the creation of forest plots. Next, an additional axis for NNT was manually added to each forest plot, as described previously by Altman.[10]

Those trials that have CIs crossing the null axis (dashed line at 0 and ∞) display insignificant results, meaning that it cannot be stated with 95% confidence that the use of that drug, in that group of cattle, had a positive effect compared with treatment with saline sham injection. Each of the antimicrobials reported with insignificant CIs in this report was shown to have substantial evidence of clinical efficacy by different statistical tests of significance, as found in each of their respective FOI summaries. And, these studies were accepted as proof of efficacy in the drug approval process. CI estimation for the comparison of 2 proportions is not without its drawbacks, including the creation of intervals that do not make logical sense, termed *aberrations*, and an achieved CI different from the intended $1-\alpha$.[9] The method used in this article, however, performs well with large sample sizes and is less affected by unequal sample sizes compared with many other methods.[11]

As discussed by Altman, trials resulting in ARR lower CIs that are negative present a problem when presenting data as the NNT. The inverse of a very small negative number is another larger negative number that is completely illogical, clinically. As an example, the reciprocal of the ARR 95% lower CI of ceftiofur sodium, 1.1 mg/kg intramuscularly daily for 3 days (DSR1 in **Fig. 6**), is −438, which by definition means that −438 animals need to be treated to have a positive outcome in 1 case. Although this makes little clinical sense, it also presents a problem when graphing these data. The solution is to think of this in terms of the drug having no effect or an infinite number of animals that could be treated without seeing a positive outcome due to the antimicrobial, seen graphically in **Figs. 6–8**.

An overwhelming majority of trials show a positive effect on case outcome in therapy for and control of BRD. The median NNT in therapeutic trials involving negative controls is 2. Therefore, for every 2 animals treated for BRD in the overall population of these studies, 1 case was a treatment success, seen in the last row of **Fig. 6** (labeled

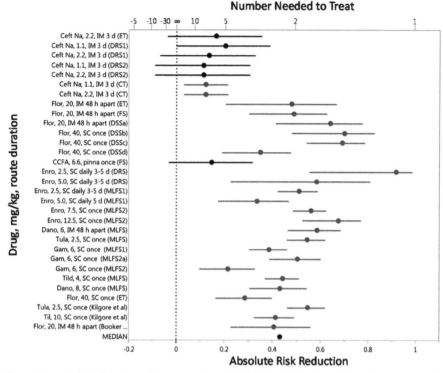

Fig. 6. Forest plot of point estimates and 95% CI of the ARR of morbidity (*bottom X axis*) and the corresponding NNT (*top X axis*) found from analysis of the therapeutic studies. Studies listed on the Y axis correspond in order to those listed in **Table 1** and are listed by active ingredient, dose (mg/kg), route of administration, and duration of therapy. CT, clinical trial.

Median). The median NNT for preventing 1 mortality due to BRD in the trials reviewed is 6; for every 6 animals treated, therapeutically, 1 BRD death is prevented (displayed in **Fig. 7**). In **Fig. 8**, for BRD control studies, the median number of animals that need to be treated to prevent 1 acute case of BRD is 5.

EXTERNAL VALIDITY OF THE INCLUDED TRIALS

A vast majority of the clinical trial data used in this review were generated in what is classified as high-risk calves, where significant morbidity is expected due to comingling and accumulated stress plus the lack of optimal vaccination or nutritional protocols in many cases. Therefore, application of these NNT values to low-risk calves, yearling cattle, or cows is inappropriate other than as a general indication of potential effects.

Other key determinants of external validity are the study entrance and success/failure criteria. These are summarized for the referenced sources of clinical trial data in **Tables 1** and **2**. The case definitions for both study entrance and success/failure vary by study. Interpretation of the criteria is also expected to vary by investigator. In the opinion of the second author, the case definitions for success required to achieve concurrence with the FDA Center for Veterinary Medicine on pivotal clinical

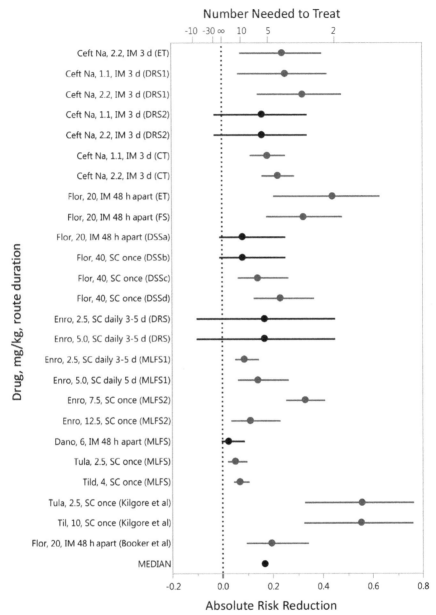

Fig. 7. Forest plot of point estimates and 95% CIs of the ARR of mortality (*bottom X axis*) and the corresponding NNT (*top X axis*) found from analysis of the therapeutic studies. Studies listed on the Y axis correspond in order to those listed in **Table 1** and are listed by active ingredient, dose (mg/kg), route of administration, and duration of therapy. CT, clinical trial.

trial protocols are likely to result in a lower success rate than criteria commonly applied in commercial settings. Although this may still result in valid testing when applied to all treatments, there is the potential for being overly conservative when estimating the effect of these antimicrobials in a commercial setting.

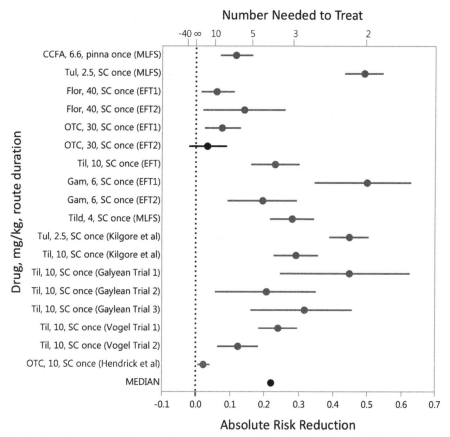

Fig. 8. Forest plot of point estimates and 95% CIs of the ARR (*bottom X axis*) and the corresponding NNT (*top X axis*) found from analysis of the control studies. Studies listed on the Y correspond in order to those listed in **Table 1** and are listed by active ingredient, dose (mg/kg), route of administration, and duration of therapy. CT, clinical trial.

DISCUSSION

The objective of this article is to explore the effectiveness of antimicrobials in therapy for and control of BRD compared with no treatment. Extreme caution should be taken in directly comparing the NNT of one antimicrobial to another due to differences in trial design, sample size discrepancies, risk classification differences of BRD between trials, resultant spontaneous recovery rates, and potential differences in case definition and success/failure outcome between trials. In the authors' opinion, because a bulk of the data come from FOI summaries, a majority of the variables (population risk status and case and success/failure definitions) are similar and provide a better means of comparison than meta-analysis of trials using positive treatment controls.

The presentation of the data in this manner also makes for a succinct way of defining reasonable expectations of efficacy in the treatment and control of BRD in a field setting for cattle at high risk of BRD. It should be pointed out again that clinicians interpreting these data need to bear in mind the external validity of these studies when applying them to the type of cattle, environmental setting, and typical BRD pathogens encountered in their practices.

REFERENCES

1. Watts JL, Sweeney MT. Antimicrobial resistance in bovine respiratory disease pathogens: measures, trends, and impact on efficacy. Vet Clin North Am Food Anim Pract 2010;26:79–88 Table of contents.
2. Cook RJ, Sackett DL. The number needed to treat: a clinically useful measure of treatment effect. BMJ 1995;310:452–4.
3. Francoz D, Buczinski S, Apley M. Evidence related to the use of ancillary drugs in bovine respiratory disease (anti-inflammatory and others): are they justified or not? Vet Clin North Am Food Anim Pract 2012;28:23–38, vii–viii.
4. O'Connor AM, Coetzee JF, da Silva N, et al. A mixed treatment comparison meta-analysis of antibiotic treatments for bovine respiratory disease. Prev Vet Med 2013;110:77–87.
5. Vogel GJ, Laudert SB, Zimmermann A, et al. Effects of tilmicosin on acute undifferentiated respiratory tract disease in newly arrived feedlot cattle. J Am Vet Med Assoc 1998;212:1919–24.
6. Hibbard B, Robb EJ, Chester ST Jr, et al. Dose determination and confirmation for ceftiofur crystalline-free acid administered in the posterior aspect of the ear for control and treatment of bovine respiratory disease. Vet Ther 2002;3:22–30.
7. Hamm M, Wollen T, Highland R, et al. Clinical efficacy of enrofloxacin against bovine respiratory disease comparing different treatment regimens. Bov Pract 1999;33:56–9.
8. Messersmith RE, Brown LN, Anderson SW, et al. Respiratory disease in recently-shipped Minnesota steers (a clinical study). Vet Med Small Anim Clin 1972;67:1011–6.
9. Newcombe RG. Interval estimation for the difference between independent proportions: comparison of eleven methods. Stat Med 1998;17:873–90.
10. Altman DG. Confidence intervals for the number needed to treat. BMJ 1998;317:1309–12.
11. Laud PJ, Dane A. Confidence intervals for the difference between independent binomial proportions: comparison using a graphical approach and moving averages. Pharm Stat 2014;13:294–308.
12. Freedom of information summary, 1998. NADA 140-338 Naxcel sterile powder - original approval. Available at: http://www.fda.gov/AnimalVeterinary/Products/ApprovedAnimalDrugProducts/FOIADrugSummaries/ucm049764.htm. Accessed August 8, 2014.
13. Freedom of information summary, 1996. NADA 141-063 Nuflor injectable solution - original approval. Available at: http://www.fda.gov/AnimalVeterinary/Products/ApprovedAnimalDrugProducts/FOIADrugSummaries/ucm116713.htm. Accessed August 8, 2014.
14. Freedom of information summary, 1998b. NADA 141-063 Nuflor injectable solution. Available at: http://www.fda.gov/downloads/AnimalVeterinary/Products/ApprovedAnimalDrugProducts/FOIADrugSummaries/ucm116741.pdf. Accessed August 8, 2014.
15. Freedom of information summary, 2003. NADA 141-209 Excede sterile suspension - original approval. Available at: http://www.fda.gov/downloads/AnimalVeterinary/Products/ApprovedAnimalDrugProducts/FOIADrugSummaries/ucm117761.pdf. Accessed August 8, 2014.
16. Freedom of information summary, 1996. NADA 141-068 Baytril 100 injectable solution - original approval. Available at: http://www.fda.gov/AnimalVeterinary/Products/ApprovedAnimalDrugProducts/FOIADrugSummaries/ucm116766.htm.

17. Freedom of information summary, 2002. NADA 141-207 A180 Sterile antimicrobial injectable solution - original approval. Available at: http://www.fda.gov/downloads/AnimalVeterinary/Products/ApprovedAnimalDrugProducts/FOIADrugSummaries/ucm117754.pdf.

18. Freedom of information summary, 2005. NADA 141-244 Draxxin Injectable Solution - original approval. Available at: http://www.fda.gov/downloads/AnimalVeterinary/Products/ApprovedAnimalDrugProducts/FOIADrugSummaries/ucm118061.pdf.

19. Freedom of information summary, 2011. NADA 141-328 Zactran injectable solution - original approval. Available at: http://www.fda.gov/downloads/AnimalVeterinary/Products/ApprovedAnimalDrugProducts/FOIADrugSummaries/UCM277806.pdf.

20. Freedom of information summary, 2012. NADA 141-334 Zuprevo injectable solution - original approval. Available at: http://www.fda.gov/downloads/AnimalVeterinary/Products/ApprovedAnimalDrugProducts/FOIADrugSummaries/UCM314826.pdf.

21. Freedom of information summary, 2011. NADA 141-207 Advocin sterile injectable solution - supplemental approval. Available at: http://www.fda.gov/downloads/AnimalVeterinary/Products/ApprovedAnimalDrugProducts/FOIADrugSummaries/UCM292024.pdf.

22. Freedom of information summary, 2009. NADA 141-265 Nuflor Gold - original approval. Available at: http://www.fda.gov/downloads/AnimalVeterinary/Products/ApprovedAnimalDrugProducts/FOIADrugSummaries/ucm062315.pdf.

23. Kilgore WR, Spensley MS, Sun F, et al. Therapeutic efficacy of tulathromycin, a novel triamilide antimicrobial, against bovine respiratory disease in feeder calves. Vet Ther 2005;6:143–53.

24. Booker CW, Jim GK, Guichon PT, et al. Evaluation of florfenicol for the treatment of undifferentiated fever in feedlot calves in western Canada. Can Vet J 1997;38:555–60.

25. Freedom of information summary, 2003. NADA 141-143 Tetradure 300 injection - original approval. Available at: http://www.fda.gov/downloads/AnimalVeterinary/Products/ApprovedAnimalDrugProducts/FOIADrugSummaries/ucm117183.pdf.

26. Freedom of information summary, 1992. NADA 140-929 Micotil 300-original approval. Available at: http://www.fda.gov/AnimalVeterinary/Products/ApprovedAnimalDrugProducts/FOIADrugSummaries/ucm054869.htm.

27. Kilgore WR, Nutsch RG, Spensley MS, et al. Clinical effectiveness of tulathromycin, a novel triamilide antimicrobial, for the control of respiratory disease in cattle at high risk for developing bovine respiratory disease. Vet Ther 2005;6:136–42.

28. Galyean ML, Gunter SA, Malcolm-Callis KJ. Effects of arrival medication with tilmicosin phosphate on health and performance of newly received beef cattle. J Anim Sci 1995;73:1219–26.

29. Johnson JC, Bryson WL, Barringer S, et al. Evaluation of on-arrival versus prompted metaphylaxis regimes using ceftiofur crystalline free acid for feedlot heifers at risk of developing bovine respiratory disease. Vet Ther 2008;9:53–62.

30. Hendrick SH, Bateman KG, Rosengren LB. The effect of antimicrobial treatment and preventive strategies on bovine respiratory disease and genetic relatedness and antimicrobial resistance of Mycoplasma bovis isolates in a western Canadian feedlot. Can Vet J 2013;54:1146–56.

Clinical Pharmacology of Analgesic Drugs in Cattle

Matthew L. Stock, VMD, Johann F. Coetzee, BVSc, Cert CHP, PhD, MRCVS*

KEYWORDS

- Local anesthetics • Nonsteroidal anti-inflammatory drugs • Opioids • α2-Agonists
- N-methyl-D-aspartate receptor antagonists • Gabapentin

KEY POINTS

- The Animal Medicinal Drug Use Clarification Act regulates the extralabel drug use of analgesics in cattle within the United States.
- Compounds including local anesthetics, nonsteroidal anti-inflammatory drugs, opioids, α2-agonists, N-methyl-D-aspartate receptor antagonists, and gabapentin are reviewed, with an emphasis on evidence of analgesia in cattle during pain states.
- Given the variety of pharmacokinetic and pharmacodynamic properties of pain-relieving drugs, evidence needs to drive the development of analgesic protocols for cattle during pain-related events.
- A multimodal approach using both local anesthesia and an anti-inflammatory drug optimizes pain relief in livestock procedures known to cause distress and pain.
- The use of meloxicam, ketoprofen, and flunixin in the development of analgesic protocols is potentially supported by randomized controlled trials.

INTRODUCTION

Pain states in cattle are common. Both iatrogenic pain attributable to livestock management procedures such as dehorning or castration and disease-associated pain including lameness, abdominal disorders, or sepsis are frequently encountered. Regardless of the origin, a noxious insult is typically translated into a chemical and electric signal, which is modulated in the dorsal horn of the spinal cord and perceived in the brain.[1,2] This initial phase is often associated with acute pain; however, a second prolonged and diffuse phase often results in local hypersensitivity.[2] Persistence of this

Dr M.L. Stock has nothing to disclose. Dr J.F. Coetzee is supported by Agriculture and Food Research Initiative Competitive Grant no. 2013-67015-21332 from the USDA National Institute of Food and Agriculture, and has been a consultant for Merck Animal Health, Norbrook Laboratories Ltd. Midwest Veterinary Services, and Boehringer Ingelheim Vetmedica.
Department of Veterinary Diagnostic and Production Animal Medicine, College of Veterinary Medicine, Iowa State University, 2448 Lloyd Vet Med, Ames, IA 50011, USA
* Corresponding author.
E-mail address: hcoetzee@iastate.edu

delayed response may cause systemic hypersensitivity known as central sensitization ("wind-up"),[2,3] clinically manifesting as hyperalgesia (ie, increased pain from a painful stimulus) and allodynia (ie, pain from a nonpainful stimulus).[4] Analgesics are provided, if possible, to mitigate both the acute and prolonged phases of pain associated with the noxious stimuli.

Pain associated with castration and dehorning results in both the described acute and delayed responses. Following the initial noxious insult either from a surgical incision (eg, scrotal incision, Barnes dehorners) or cautery dehorning, stress as determined by cortisol concentrations peaks approximately 30 minutes after the procedure.[5,6] Subsequently a delayed response occurs, as evidenced by increased sensitivity and behavioral, physiologic, and immunologic changes that may persist for up to 44 hours.[7–9] Recent studies suggest that dehorning results in a more acute stress response in comparison with castration as evidenced by cortisol concentrations obtained under the same experimental conditions.[10,11] Furthermore, dehorning 2 to 3 weeks postcastration resulted in an increased stress response and decreased average daily gain (ADG) in comparison with animals that were dehorned first and castrated later.[12] Conversely, castration in cattle resulted in an amplified immune response when compared with dehorning in the same study, suggesting more of an inflammatory effect.[10] When dehorning and castration were combined, the acute cortisol changes were additive, whereas the immune changes were not.[10,11]

Lameness is a disease that may be recognized during an acute or chronic phase. Progression of acute pain to chronic disease may result in neurologic changes, making individuals refractory to analgesic treatment.[13] As such, naturally occurring lameness may represent issues concerning chronic pain whereby treatment failures are common because of the complexity of neuropathic pain development.[13] Drugs targeting neuropathic pain such as gabapentin may be useful for analgesic treatment in these cases of chronic pain.

Providing analgesia to cattle is not without its challenges. Primarily, from a regulatory perspective no analgesic drugs are specifically approved for the alleviation of pain in livestock.[14] The Animal Medicinal Drug Use Clarification Act (AMDUCA) of 1994 permits extralabel drug use (ELDU) to relieve suffering in cattle.[15] As such, analgesics would be permitted under AMDUCA given that the criteria for ELDU are followed. In addition to these regulations, pain medications can be costly, difficult to administer, and short-acting, requiring frequent administration, and may be controlled substances necessitating a veterinary license.[7] Moreover, cattle do not overtly demonstrate signs of pain, making it difficult for some producers to observe the value in providing pain relief, especially given a lack of support for economic gain.[7]

Despite these challenges, analgesics have demonstrated numerous benefits to cattle during pain states. Following castration, analgesics have reduced the physiologic, behavioral, and neuroendocrine changes that occur following the noxious stimuli (**Figs. 1** and **2**).[16] These changes are also observed in cattle after dehorning or disbudding using analgesics (**Figs. 3** and **4**).[8,17] Lameness models have demonstrated improvements following administration of NSAIDs as detected by pressure mats; however the use of NSAIDs have provided minimal analgesic effects in naturally occurring lameness as determined by locomotion scoring (**Fig. 5**).[18–21] This may be a result of the differences associated with acute and chronic pain states or potentially due to an increase sensitivity of pressure mats to detect differences between lame cattle. Perhaps a more compelling motivation for the use of analgesia in cattle may concern the relationship between the autonomic nervous system and the immune response. Activation of the sympathetic nervous system has demonstrated immunosuppressive effects that may incite and progress systemic infections.[22] Although this

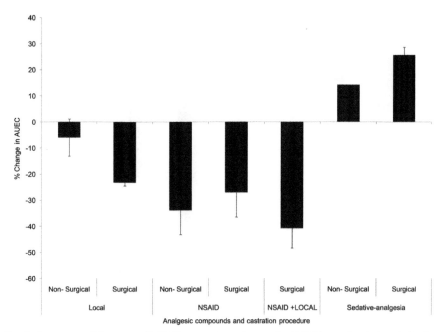

Fig. 1. Summary of the mean (±SEM) percentage change in AUEC in analgesic-treated calves compared with untreated castrated control calves in the published literature. Percentage change in cortisol was calculated using the formula [(Mean of analgesic group/Mean of castrated control group) − 1] × 100. (*From* Coetzee JF. Assessment and management of pain associated with castration in cattle. Vet Clin North Am Food Anim Pract 2013;29:92; with permission.)

relationship has not been elucidated in cattle, it may offer an explanation of the reduced pull rate and bovine respiratory disease morbidity in cattle receiving meloxicam following castration on arrival at a feedlot.[23]

Previous comprehensive reviews of the literature have reported that effective analgesia in cattle is achieved through a multimodal approach (**Figs. 1–4**).[6,17,24] Administering different pharmaceuticals to antagonize or attenuate the transmission, modulation, and perception of the pain signal optimizes pain relief (**Fig. 6**).[1] Furthermore, the provision of a combination of compounds with different onsets and duration of action addresses both the acute and delayed phases of pain. With a multimodal approach, effective drug concentrations may be optimized to coincide with the occurrence of pain. Analgesia is maximized by combining local anesthesia, nonsteroidal anti-inflammatory drugs (NSAIDs), opioids, α2-agonists, N-methyl-D-aspartate (NMDA) receptor antagonists, and neuropathic pain antagonists. These analgesic options are reviewed herein in regard to clinical pharmacology, with special attention on evidence-based compounds investigated with randomized, placebo-controlled trials (RCTs). It is notable that trial masking was not considered for inclusion in this review. Of the 19 dehorning studies included in the summary graphs (see **Figs. 3** and **4**), 7 trials were explicitly stated as masked. Moreover, the 5 lameness studies used to construct the summary data (see **Fig. 5**) were all explicitly stated as being masked. The castration graphs (see **Figs. 1** and **2**) were published in a previous edition of *Veterinary Clinics of North America Food Animal Practice*, derived from data whereby masking was not recorded.[24] Additional discussion of studies with an undocumented masking status have been included in this review as descriptive data.

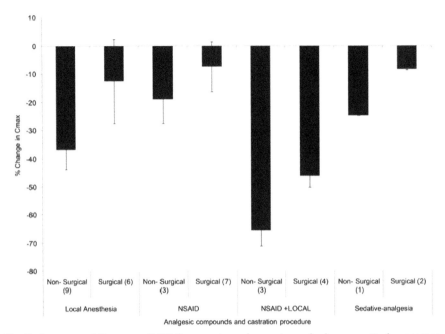

Fig. 2. Summary of the mean (±SEM) percentage change in peak plasma cortisol concentrations (Cmax) in analgesic-treated calves compared with untreated castrated control calves in the published literature. The number of treatment groups evaluated is indicated in parentheses. Percentage change in cortisol was calculated using the formula [(Mean of analgesic group/Mean of castrated control group) − 1] × 100. (*From* Coetzee JF. Assessment and management of pain associated with castration in cattle. Vet Clin North Am Food Anim Pract 2013;29:91; with permission.)

LOCAL ANESTHESIA

The most commonly used analgesics in cattle are local anesthetics. By blocking sodium channels within nerve cells, the conduction and transmission of the pain signal is inhibited.[25] As such, the region where the anesthetic is deposited is devoid of sensation. Of benefit to the patient experiencing a noxious stimulus, stimulated nerves are more sensitive to local anesthesia. Moreover, nerves responsible for pain and temperature are blocked before those fibers involved with touch, pressure, and motor activity.[26]

Although the observed effect is reversible, its duration of action depends on the length of contact time with the nerve.[26] Therefore, innate chemical properties that determine rates of absorption and tissue distribution, as well as metabolism, are heavily involved in determining the length of desensitization. Moreover, the addition of vasoconstrictor compounds (eg, epinephrine) to increase contact time through reduction of both absorption and metabolism may be beneficial.[26] However, as local environment is crucial to the activity of a local anesthetic, infected tissues with a decreased pH may reduce the effect.

Several administration routes are available for local anesthetics, including injection via a needle, needle-free techniques, and topical. When injected, the onset of activity for lidocaine is fairly rapid, occurring within 2 to 5 minutes and persisting for approximately 90 minutes.[7] This duration is prolonged (median 304 minutes; range: 107–512 minutes) with the addition of epinephrine (0.01 mg/mL).[27] Additional injectable anesthetics such as bupivacaine may provide superior duration of activity (5–8 hours);

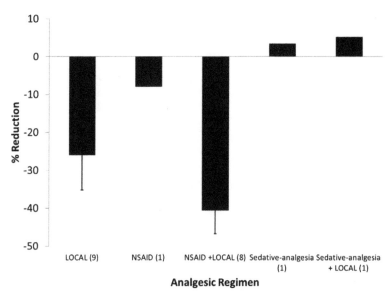

Analgesic Regimen

Fig. 3. Mean (±SEM) percentage reduction in the area under the plasma cortisol concentration over time curve (AUEC) or overall mean cortisol concentrations following dehorning using analgesia. The number of treatment groups evaluated is indicated in parentheses. Percentage change in cortisol was calculated using the formula [(Mean of analgesic group/Mean of control group) − 1] × 100. (*Data from* Stock ML, Baldridge SL, Griffin D, et al. Bovine dehorning: assessing pain and providing analgesic management. Vet Clin North Am Food Anim Pract 2013;29:103–33.)

however, onset may be delayed (20–30 minutes).[25] Recently, a gel-based topical local anesthetic consisting of lidocaine, bupivacaine, adrenaline (epinephrine), and cetrimide (Tri-Solfen; Bayer Animal Health, Australia) demonstrated rapid desensitization of scrotal mucosal tissue with effects lasting 24 hours.[28] Regional anesthesia via epidural administration of lidocaine (0.2 mg/kg) produces fairly rapid (5 minutes) desensitization of the perineal region for a time interval of 10 to 115 minutes.[29]

Castration

Local anesthesia is beneficial to cattle during the acute pain phase associated with castration. In a review of 15 castration studies evaluating maximum cortisol concentrations of calves treated only with a local anesthetic, cortisol was reduced by an average 25.8% (95% confidence interval [CI] 2.46%–49.1%) compared with control calves.[24] This magnitude of effect was not as large when evaluating the integrated cortisol response throughout the study period (area under the effect curve [AUEC]).[24] Prior evidence suggests that administration of a local anesthetic alone has minimal effect on overall feed consumption, ADG, and inflammatory mediators.[30–33] However, a recent study evaluated the effect of a combined lidocaine/bupivacaine product with a vasoconstrictor and antiseptic (Tri-Solfen) applied to the exposed mucosal surfaces of the spermatic cord and surgical incision administered alone.[28] In this prospective masked controlled trial, treated calves demonstrated reduced pain-related behaviors and tolerated more pressure at both the castration site and surrounding skin for 24 hours after the procedure.[28] Lomax and Windsor[28] hypothesized that the rapid absorption and superior effects of the lidocaine/bupivacaine combination may aid in the prevention of central sensitization. Moreover, the

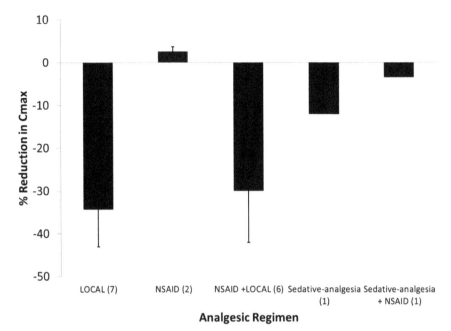

Fig. 4. Mean (±SEM) percentage reduction in peak plasma cortisol concentrations following dehorning using analgesia. The number of treatment groups evaluated is indicated in parentheses. Percentage change in cortisol was calculated using the formula [(Mean of analgesic group/Mean of control group) − 1] × 100. (*Data from* Stock ML, Baldridge SL, Griffin D, et al. Bovine dehorning: assessing pain and providing analgesic management. Vet Clin North Am Food Anim Pract 2013;29:103–33.)

adrenaline (epinephrine) may reduce the amplification of the immune response through vasoconstriction, thereby decreasing inflammatory mediators at the injury site that can result in hyperalgesia.[34]

Dehorning

The effects of a local anesthesia in dehorning or disbudding studies are similar to those in castration. The acute pain and stress associated with dehorning is attenuated in comparison with untreated controls as determined by cortisol concentrations.[6,17] This effect is primarily observed for the duration of the local anesthetic activity for up to 5 hours after dehorning.[17] Moreover, evaluation of the autonomic nervous system through heart rate variability and ocular temperatures indicate an imbalance 2 to 3 hours after dehorning with lidocaine administration, coinciding with the time associated with loss of lidocaine activity.[35] Of note, ADG,[36] heart rate,[36] immune function,[37] and lying time[38] are minimally affected by administration of only a local anesthetic.

It is interesting that the method of administration prolongs the local desensitization in dehorning anesthesia.[27] An approximately 2.5-hour median duration increase was reported following a cornual nerve block when compared with a ring block using lidocaine and epinephrine in combination.[27]

Lameness

Anesthesia of the lower limb and foot is most often performed using intravenous regional anesthesia or a ring block with lidocaine. Typically this procedure facilitates diagnostics or treatment of an injured distal limb for the duration a tourniquet remains

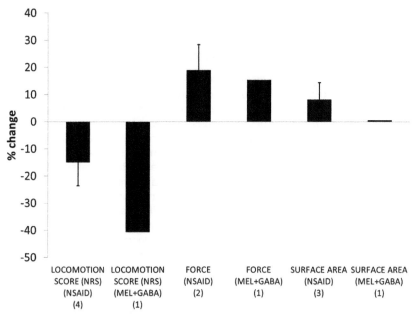

Fig. 5. Mean (±SEM) percentage change of response variables during the treatment of naturally occurring or induced lameness using an NSAID alone or with gabapentin (MEL+′″ GABA). Number in parentheses indicates studies reviewed. Percentage change in response variable was calculated using the formula [(Mean of analgesic group/Mean of control group) − 1] × 100.

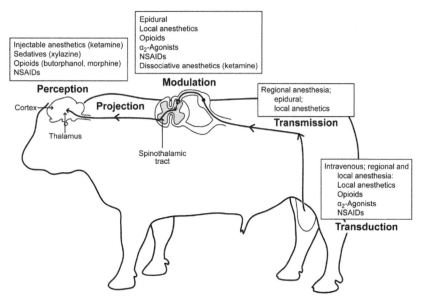

Fig. 6. The nociceptive pathway in cattle, indicating the anatomic location of target receptors for analgesic drug activity. (*From* Coetzee JF. A review of analgesic compounds used in food animals in the United States. Vet Clin North Am Food Anim Pract 2013;29:13; with permission.)

in place.[39] Because of the required skill and labor, and the short duration of effect, lidocaine is rarely used as a stand-alone treatment for lameness.

NONSTEROIDAL ANTI-INFLAMMATORY DRUGS

NSAIDs primarily inhibit cyclooxygenase (COX) isoenzymes, subsequently reducing the production of prostaglandins (PG) from arachidonic acid.[4] In addition to contributing to the inflammatory response through vasodilation and inflammatory cell recruitment, PG in concert with other cytokines and neuropeptides decreases the action potential threshold in nociceptors and propagates the pain signal.[40] Peripherally this causes a local hyperalgesia or peripheral sensitization. Moreover, COX isoenzymes present in the spinal cord produce excess PG following acute noxious stimuli, leading to central sensitization and chronic pain,[40] clinically indicated by hyperalgesia and allodynia. Both isoenzymes COX-1 and COX-2 are thought to be responsible for the inflammatory response, with the initial effects a result of COX-1–derived PG and the delayed effects attributable to upregulation of COX-2 expression.[41] As such, NSAIDs that target both isoenzymes may be advantageous for both immediate and prolonged pain; however, increased inhibition of COX-1 is associated with adverse renal and gastrointestinal effects.[40]

NSAIDs are typically weak acids with a low pK_a, resulting in good oral bioavailability in monogastrics.[25] With the exception of firocoxib, NSAIDs commonly used in veterinary species generally have a low volume of distribution, most likely attributable to the high plasma protein binding, which may affect overall tissue distribution.[42] Elimination can occur through the renal system following metabolism in the liver; however, reports of biliary secretion leading to fecal elimination is observed in other species.[42,43] Compounds known as COX-2 selective or COX-1 sparing were developed to reduce the potential for adverse effects associated with COX-1 inhibition. These molecules were designed with side chains too large to bind to the smaller COX-1 active site, and therefore are only physically able to bind COX-2.[40] **Table 1** summarizes the unique properties and pharmacokinetics of NSAIDs available in the United States.

An extensive review of the literature suggests, in general, that NSAIDs mitigate the overall AUEC cortisol response by a greater magnitude than their ability to reduce peak cortisol concentrations following castration and dehorning (see **Figs. 1–4**).[17,24] Moreover, NSAIDs alone may not be adequate to control the associated distress after dehorning (see **Figs. 3** and **4**); although this conclusion should be interpreted with caution as it is drawn from a small number of studies. The analgesic effect of NSAIDs is amplified with the use of a local anesthetic for both castration and dehorning (see **Figs. 1–4**). Primarily, NSAIDs provide analgesia during the delayed phase of pain observed postoperatively in both castration and dehorning procedures.

Flunixin Meglumine

Derived from nicotinic acid in the anthranilic acid NSAID class, Flunixin is the only NSAID approved by the Food and Drug Administration (FDA) for cattle in the United States.[14] At present, flunixin is indicated for the control of fever associated with respiratory disease or mastitis, and fever and inflammation associated with endotoxemia. Pharmacokinetic properties are presented in **Table 1**. Given its anti-inflammatory properties, it has been evaluated as a pain reliever.

Castration

Investigations into the analgesic effects of flunixin indicate pain relief during the initial period postcastration. Cortisol concentrations obtained 6 hours after burdizzo-clamp castrations were significantly less in calves treated with flunixin meglumine (2.2 mg/kg) and a lidocaine epidural in comparison with untreated controls.[44] Attenuation of the

Table 1
Analgesic compounds available for use in cattle

Drug	Approved Species	Indications	Dose (mg/kg)	Route	$T_{1/2}$	F (%)	T_{max}	Withhold Time	Comments
NSAID									
Flunixin meglumine	Cattle, horses, pigs	Antipyretic, anti-inflammatory	2.2 2.2	IV PO	3–8 h 6.2 h	60	3.5 ± 1.0 h	Meat: 4 d Milk: 36 h Not approved route for cattle	IV only approved route PO/IM: prolonged withhold IM: tissue necrosis
Phenylbutazone	Horses, dogs	Anti-inflammatory	4 4–8	IV only! PO	40–55 h 57.9 ± 6.5 h	54–69	8.9–11.7 h	Not approved for cattle in the USA	ELDU prohibited for dairy cattle ≥20 mo Use strongly discouraged
Ketoprofen	Horses, dogs; EU approval in EU and Canada	Anti-inflammatory; adjunctive therapy for fever, pain, and inflammation associated with mastitis (EU)	3	IV, IM	0.42 h			Not approved for cattle in the USA	Concentrates in inflammatory exudates Consists of racemic RS± enantiomers S(+) >R(−) inhibiting PGE_2 Multiple doses may be required to maintain analgesia
Aspirin/sodium salicylate	No formal FDA approval for cattle and horses	Reduction of fever Relief of minor muscle aches and joint pain	50–100	PO IV	3.7 ± 0.4 h 0.5 h	<20		No formal FDA approval Not for use in lactating cattle	PO: rumen acts as reservoir for slow absorption Limited tissue distribution (low V_d) Not associated with clotting deficits in cattle

(continued on next page)

Table 1
(continued)

Drug	Approved Species	Indications	Dose (mg/kg)	Route	$T_{1/2}$	F (%)	T_{max}	Withhold Time	Comments
Carprofen	Dogs; EU approval for cattle	Anti-inflammatory, antipyretic; adjunctive therapy for acute respiratory disease and mastitis	1.4	IV, SC	<10 wk: R(−): 49.7 ± 3.9 h; S(+): 37.4 ± 2.4 h; Adult: RS±: 30.7±2.3 h			Not approved for cattle in the USA	Consists of racemic RS± enantiomers S(+) > R(−) inhibiting PGE2
Meloxicam	Dogs and cats; EU and Canadian approval for cattle	Adjunctive therapy for acute respiratory disease; diarrhea and acute mastitis; pain associated with dehorning (Canada)	0.5 / 0.5–1.0	IV, SC / PO	22 ± 3 h / 27 h (20–43 h)	100	11.6 h	Not approved in cattle in the USA	Both injectable and oral tablet formulations available
Firocoxib	Horses, dogs	Anti-inflammatory	0.5	PO	18.8 h (14.2–25.5 h)	98	4 h	Not approved for cattle in the USA	Evaluated in preweaned calves
Opioid									
Butorphanol	Dogs, cats, horses	Analgesia; sedation	0.025	IM	71 ± 8 min		9.5 ± 0.5 min	Not approved for cattle in the USA	PK data following coadministration with ketamine and xylazine
Nalbuphine	No known veterinary-labeled product	Analgesia	0.4	IV	41 min (32–47 min)			Not approved in cattle in the USA	Plasma samples undetectable after 3 h

α2-Agonist

Drug	Species	Indication	Dose	Route	$T_{1/2}$		Approval	Comments
Xylazine	Dogs, cats, horses, deer, elk; EU approval for cattle	Sedation; analgesia	0.05–0.3	IM	96 ± 20 min	9.5 ± 0.5 min	Not approved for cattle in the USA	PK data following coadministration with ketamine and butorphanol; Dose-dependent response: higher doses result in recumbency; Fast to prevent rumen tympany; aspiration of rumen contents

NMDA antagonist

| Ketamine | Cats | Sedation; analgesia | 0.1 | IM
IV | 67 ± 11 min
29.4 ± 4.5 min | 10 ± 1 min | Not approved for cattle in the USA | PK data following coadministration with xylazine alone (IV) or with xylazine and butorphanol (IM); Metabolite norketamine may contribute to analgesia |

Neuropathic pain analgesic

| Gabapentin | No known veterinary-labeled product | Neuropathic analgesia | 15 | PO | 7.9 h (6.9–12.4 h) | 7.2 h (6–10 h) | Not approved for cattle in the USA | Plasma concentrations above those reported as therapeutic in humans for up to 15 hrs |

Abbreviations: ELDU, extralabel drug use; EU, European Union; F, bioavailability; FDA, US Food and Drug Administration; IM, intramuscular; IV, intravenous; PGE$_2$, prostaglandin E$_2$; PO, per os (oral); SC, subcutaneous; T$_{1/2}$, elimination half-life; V$_d$, volume of distribution; PK, pharmacokinetic.

mean peak cortisol concentration after surgical castration following flunixin (2 mg/kg; intramuscular) administration was also observed compared with castrated controls.[10] Webster and colleagues[30] demonstrated similar reductions of the integrated and peak cortisol concentrations in 2- to 3-month-old calves administered intravenous flunixin (1.1 mg/kg) in combination with local anesthesia before castration when compared with placebo-treated controls. In addition to cortisol, stride length is reported to increase in calves treated with flunixin (2.2 mg/kg) in combination with a lidocaine epidural for up to 8 hours after surgical castration in comparison with control calves.[45] These changes in stride length and increased feed intake were also observed in band castrated calves treated with intravenous flunixin (1.1 mg/kg) in combination with a xylazine epidural.[46] Flunixin meglumine (2 mg/kg; intramuscular) combined with local anesthesia was protective against the leukocytosis, neutrophilia, and increased haptoglobin observed in untreated controls following surgical castration.[10] Flunixin administration is associated with pain relief, although, in general, these reported changes are not reported to persist beyond 8 hours.

Dehorning
Flunixin administration provided benefits to calves during the acute stress and painful phase following dehorning. Flunixin meglumine (2 mg/kg) administered to calves following a cornual nerve block reduced cortisol concentrations for 3 and 6 hours in comparison with untreated controls in calves undergoing chemical[47] and amputation dehorning,[10] respectively. Moreover, in addition to a local anesthetic, flunixin (2.2 mg/kg) administered to calves preoperatively and again 3 hours after cautery dehorning had a significantly reduced integrated cortisol concentration over an 8-hour study period with significant reductions at 0.5 and 2 hours when compared with dehorned controls.[48] However, heart and respiratory rates were unaffected. The alleviation of the initial pain response is consistent with flunixin concentrations that suppress ex vivo prostaglandin E_2 (PGE_2) concentrations for up to 12 hours in calves surgically dehorned.[49]

In addition to analgesic effects observed in the acute pain period, cortisol concentrations and average daily gains were significantly improved over 7 days for calves treated with flunixin (2.2 mg/kg) compared with untreated calves.[50] With intravenous administration, analgesic concentrations may have been rapidly achieved, potentially reducing central sensitization; however, evidence for this in cattle is scarce.[51] One study reported equivocal analgesic response in calves receiving an NSAID 12 hours prior versus immediately before dehorning, indicating the pain response was not alleviated with preemptive analgesia.[52] Of interest, flunixin (2 mg/kg) combined with a cornual nerve block was protective against the observed leukocytosis after amputation dehorning for up to 24 hours, compared with untreated controls.[10] The persistence of effect may be due to an intramuscular route of administration or a result of a hysteretic response of certain immune mediators.

Lameness
In both naturally occurring lameness and an amphotericin B lameness-induced model, flunixin provided acute analgesic relief to cattle. Cortisol concentrations tended to be reduced in calves treated twice with flunixin (1 mg/kg), initially at the time of lameness induction and 12 hours later, compared with placebo-treated controls.[53] Furthermore, gait changes measured on a pressure mat indicated an increased force on the ipsilateral limb in addition to decreased lying time during the first day following lameness induction.[53] In addition, an observed increase in lying time "following hoof trimming" was less prolonged in lame cattle treated with flunixin (2.2 mg/kg) daily for 2 days when compared with placebo-treated controls.[20]

Ketoprofen

Ketoprofen, an NSAID of the propionic acid class, has approval in the European Union and Canada as an adjunctive therapy for fever, pain, and inflammation associated with mastitis, and inflammatory and painful conditions of bones and joints.[54] Pharmacokinetic properties are presented in **Table 1**. Ketoprofen is administered as a racemic mixture (50:50) with chiral RS± enantiomers. Of note, the R(−) enantiomer will undergo chiral inversion to S(+), which is clinically relevant because the S(+) enantiomer is a more potent PGE_2 inhibitor.[55] Given the short half-life owing to rapid metabolism and elimination, efforts to sustain analgesia may require multiple doses. Nevertheless, many studies have investigated the analgesic potential of ketoprofen.

Castration

In both surgically and nonsurgically castrated cattle, preoperatively ketoprofen (3 mg/kg) administered in single or multiple doses demonstrated reduced peak and integrated cortisol concentrations in comparison with castrated controls.[31–33,56] This effect was potentiated when combined with a local anesthetic.[24] Feed intake is not different between ketoprofen-treated and control calves, whereas average daily gain is improved by the administration of ketoprofen (3 mg/kg) combined with a lidocaine local anesthetic for surgical[31] but not nonsurgical castration.[32] Taken together with the cortisol data, when using ketoprofen, multimodal therapy is needed for maximizing pain relief during castration.

Dehorning

Similarly to castration, ketoprofen (3 mg/kg) administration in combination with a local anesthetic resulted in the amelioration of the acute cortisol response, with effects persisting up to 5 hours in comparison with untreated controls.[57–60] With ketoprofen (3 mg/kg) administration without local anesthesia, the typically observed cortisol plateau was attenuated; however, peak cortisol concentrations were only mildly reduced.[57] A tendency for improved weight gains following multiple doses and increased starter consumption has also been reported over a 24-hour period in ketoprofen-treated calves compared with control calves,[60,61] although it is noteworthy that the analgesic regimen in these trials also included local anesthesia[60,61] and xylazine[61] for all calves dehorned.

Lameness

Ketoprofen (3 mg/kg) improved naturally occurring lameness in adult dairy cattle, based on maintenance of weight distribution using a weighing platform and locomotion scores using a 5-point numerical rating scale.[19,62] This analgesic effect was not observed at lower ketoprofen (0.3 mg/kg) doses, demonstrating dose-responsive analgesia.[19] Ketoprofen (3 mg/kg) administered once daily for 3 days also reduced the sensitivity associated with naturally occurring lameness in adult dairy cattle in comparison with placebo-treated controls.[18] This trend was evidenced by an improved nociception threshold tested at 3, 8, and 28 days after enrollment observed in the ketoprofen-treated cattle but not in cows treated with saline. As such, a 3-day intramuscular ketoprofen (3 mg/kg) regimen may help alleviate the development of hyperalgesia associated with lameness.[18]

Surgery

Newby and colleagues[63] evaluated the use of ketoprofen (3 mg/kg) administered initially at the time of left displaced abomasum surgery and once the following day. No differences were reported in response variables including heart rate, respiratory rate, β-hydroxybutyrate, and milk production, between cattle receiving either ketoprofen or saline.[63]

Salicylic Acid Derivatives

Both aspirin (acetylsalicylic acid) and sodium salicylate have historically been used in cattle as anti-inflammatory, antipyretic, and analgesic agents. Despite its common use and label claims, the FDA Center for Veterinary Medicine has never formally approved the drug.[54] As such, the use of salicylic acid derivatives should be used with caution because of the lack of tissue residue studies providing withdrawal intervals. The pharmacokinetics of salicylic acid derivatives (see **Table 1**) are associated with limited tissue distribution, slow oral absorption, and rapid elimination.[64] Given the availability and previous practices, studies have evaluated its use as an analgesic.

Castration

Cortisol concentrations were attenuated in cattle administered intravenous sodium salicylate (50 mg/kg) in a comparison with untreated controls for the first 2 hours after castration.[65] This response was correlated with salicylate compounds greater than 25 µg/mL in the treated animals.[65] Conversely, oral aspirin (50 mg/kg) did not produce analgesia evidence by the cortisol response and supported by a drug concentration not achieving the analgesic threshold.[65] This lack of response may be due to the dose used, as a previous pharmacokinetic study reported salicylate concentrations remaining higher than 30 µg/mL for 1 to 5 hours following an oral dose of 100 mg/kg.[66]

Castration and dehorning

Sodium salicylate metered in water (2.5–5 mg/mL) initiated 3 days before castration and dehorning of calves, and continued for 2 more days, resulted in improved ADGs for 13 days in addition to decreased integrated cortisol concentrations from 1 to 6 hours postprocedure compared with untreated controls.[67] These acute stress-reduction effects did not persist past 6 hours; however, ADG was increased over a 13-day period.[67] It is noteworthy that water palatability may have been affected as cattle receiving salicylate decreased the amount of water consumed.

Lameness

Based on the successful pain management of 2 cows with a nonsuppurative tarsitis, administration of oral aspirin (100 mg/kg) every 12 hours was recommended; however, this recommendation does not extend to suppurative tarsitis because of the observed treatment failure in one bull.[66] In an amphotericin B–induced lameness model evaluated in 4- to 6-month-old beef calves, sodium salicylate (50 mg/kg) administration was not associated with analgesia when compared with placebo-treated controls.[68]

Carprofen

Similar to ketoprofen, carprofen is an NSAID in the propionic acid class.[51] Both NSAIDs are administered as a racemic (50:50) mixture of RS± enantiomers; however, carprofen is not known to undergo chiral inversion.[69] For cattle in the European Union, carprofen is indicated as an adjunct to antimicrobial therapy associated with respiratory disease and mastitis. Prior pharmacodynamic studies evaluating analgesia in an inflammatory model in nonruminants indicated carprofen to have a greater anti-inflammatory and analgesic potential in comparison with phenylbutazone and aspirin.[70] Pharmacokinetics are presented in **Table 1**. Unique pharmacokinetic properties of carprofen in cattle include a prolonged half-life, slow clearance, and possible biliary drug secretion as observed in dogs.[43] Of interest is that the pharmacokinetics of carprofen are age dependent, with a prolonged half-life in younger animals

(<10 weeks) most likely attributable to the decreased clearance common to neonates.[69]

Castration

A significant reduction in cortisol concentrations was observed during a 48-hour period in calves treated with carprofen (1.4 mg/kg) combined with a lidocaine epidural, when compared with untreated castrated controls following nonsurgical clamp castration.[44] Although reductions in peak cortisol concentrations in 5.5-month-old dairy calves treated with carprofen undergoing nonsurgical castration was observed, these effects were not significant.[71] In the same study, perioperative carprofen administration reduced haptoglobin concentrations; however, rectal temperature and fibrinogen were unaffected in comparison with untreated castrated control calves.[71]

More recently, inflammatory cytokines were investigated in 5.5-month-old dairy calves undergoing nonsurgical castration (ie, band or clamp).[72] Although no treatment differences were observed in mRNA cytokine expression for interleukin (IL)-1, IL-8, IL-10, and interferon-γ, IL-6, a pro- and anti-inflammatory cytokine, was upregulated in carprofen-treated calves following clamp castration in a comparison with clamp-castrated controls. The investigators state that although this may be associated with lower cortisol concentrations in calves treated with carprofen, it more likely reflects a complicated "cytokine-endocrinological network."[72]

Dehorning

Stilwell and colleagues[73] reported that carprofen (1.4 mg/kg) in combination with a lidocaine block administered 15 minutes before cautery disbudding resulted in an attenuation of the acute cortisol concentration at 1 hour after disbudding in comparison with placebo-treated calves. However, this reduction of cortisol was transient, as untreated controls had reduced cortisol at 24 hours compared with calves receiving carprofen.[73] An RCT study conducted by the authors' group evaluating 6- to 8-week-old calves either sham dehorned or cautery dehorned following administration of carprofen (1.4 mg/kg) subcutaneously or orally, or a placebo did not indicate overall group treatment differences in measured analgesic response variables including substance P, mechanical nociception threshold, and ocular temperature.[74] However, calves receiving carprofen, regardless of route, tended to have reduced maximum cortisol concentrations and a tendency to tolerate more pressure around the horn bud for the 96-hour study duration in comparison with placebo-treated controls.[74]

Lameness

At the time of writing, the authors have been unable to locate any studies evaluating carprofen in cattle for controlling pain involved in lameness.

Meloxicam

Meloxicam is a member of the oxicam class of NSAIDs. It has approval for use in the European Union and Canada for adjunctive therapy for acute respiratory disease, diarrhea, and acute mastitis, and as an analgesic to relieve pain following dehorning in calves. Moreover, meloxicam is approved in the United States for the control pain associated with osteoarthritis in humans, dogs, and cats. The pharmacokinetics of meloxicam are presented in **Table 1**. Of note, the pharmacokinetics of meloxicam in cattle indicate a prolonged half-life and a high bioavailability when administered orally.[75] Because of these favorable properties for providing practical analgesia in cattle, many studies have recently investigated oral meloxicam as an analgesic.

Castration

Recently, meloxicam has been evaluated in cattle surgically and nonsurgically castrated. Following arrival at a feedlot, administration of meloxicam (1 mg/kg) before surgical castration to 8- to 10-month-old cattle resulted in a decreased pull rate and nearly 50% reduction in respiratory disease treatment rate compared with placebo-treated controls.[23] By contrast, providing meloxicam (0.5–1 mg/kg) daily for 3 days, whereby band castration was conducted on day 2, yielded no additional benefit in regard to performance or physiology and behavior responses in comparison with placebo-treated castrated controls.[76]

Dehorning

Several recent studies have provided support for the analgesic effect of meloxicam in cattle after dehorning or disbudding. Significant reductions in cortisol concentrations have been reported in cattle receiving a local anesthetic in combination with intramuscular meloxicam (0.5 mg/kg) compared with placebo-treated cattle receiving only a lidocaine cornual nerve block.[77] This effect persisted for up to 6 hours after cautery dehorning.[77] By contrast, another study reported no effects on cortisol concentrations following administration of only intravenous meloxicam (0.5 mg/kg) in comparison with placebo-treated controls immediately before surgical dehorning.[78] These data provide additional support for the use of a multimodal approach to reduce the distress associated with dehorning. Furthermore, physiologic variables including heart rate,[77,78] respiratory rate,[77] and time spent standing[79] were elevated in placebo-treated calves and compared with these variables in calves administered meloxicam. Maintenance of the autonomic nervous system, including heart rate variability and reduced changes to ocular temperature, was observed in 4- to 5-week-old dairy calves receiving intravenous meloxicam (0.5 mg/kg) compared with placebo following cautery dehorning.[35] In addition, placebo-treated calves are reported to be nearly twice as sensitive after cautery disbudding compared with calves treated with intramuscular meloxicam (0.5 mg/kg).[9] A reported reduction in substance P, a pain neurotransmitter, provides further support for the reduced pain sensitivity following scoop dehorning in 4-month-old calves treated with intravenous meloxicam (0.5 mg/kg) compared with untreated controls. Production parameters are also improved in meloxicam-treated cattle in comparison with placebo-treated controls, with an increased ADG[78] potentially attributable to increased feed consumption or time spent near the feeder.[9,79] In summary, intravenous or intramuscular meloxicam (0.5 mg/kg) may effectively attenuate dehorning pain and stress.

More recently, oral meloxicam (1.0 mg/kg) has been evaluated in 8- to 10-week-old calves at the time of cautery dehorning, demonstrating reduced cortisol at 4 hours and substance P at 120 hours compared with placebo-treated controls.[52] Furthermore, 6-month-old calves undergoing amputation dehorning demonstrated improved ADG when treated with oral meloxicam (1.0 mg/kg) compared with placebo-treated controls.[50] However, pain sensitivity, ocular temperature, and haptoglobin were not affected.[50,52] Oral meloxicam administration may exert a persistent analgesic effect, as evidenced by concentrations significantly inhibiting ex vivo production of PGE_2 for 48 hours compared with placebo-treated controls.[52] This effect is more prolonged when meloxicam is administered at the time of dehorning in comparison with 12 hours prior.[52]

Lameness

Following induction of an amphotericin B lameness model in 4- to 6-month-old calves, oral meloxicam (0.5 mg/kg) administered once daily for 4 days ameliorated indications of pain.[21] In addition to an increased step count in meloxicam-treated animals compared with placebo-treated controls, meloxicam concentrations were inversely associated with lameness scores and positively associated with pressure and contact of the ipsilateral limb.[21] In another RCT, Offinger and colleagues[80] evaluated intravenous meloxicam (0.5 mg/kg) administered before surgery and daily for 4 days postoperatively following resection of a naturally occurring septic distal interphalangeal joint. Meloxicam treatment improved both physiologic responses (cortisol, body temperature) and mechanical responses (lameness scores, time standing, steps taken).

Surgery
An investigation into the pain associated with a left-sided 2-step rumenotomy indicated that the first step was the most painful as evidenced by an increase in heart rate, respiratory rate, and time spent lying on the contralateral side.[81] Cows administered meloxicam (0.5 mg/kg) once consumed more feed but spent less time lying on the ipsilateral side of the incision in comparison with cows receiving ketoprofen (3 mg/kg) daily for 2 days.[81]

Mastitis
The analgesic potential of meloxicam (0.5 mg/kg) in a lipopolysaccharide-induced clinical mastitis model was investigated.[82] This study reported increased pain sensitivity at 6 hours postinduction for placebo-treated cattle compared with meloxicam-treated cattle as measured by the nociception threshold difference between the infected quarter and the other 3 noninfected quarters.[82]

Firocoxib

Firocoxib is an NSAID of the coxib class. This newer group of NSAIDs demonstrates COX-2 selectivity in dogs and horses, thereby potentially limiting adverse effects caused by COX-1 inhibition.[42] At present, in the United States firocoxib is indicated for the treatment of pain and inflammation associated with osteoarthritis in dogs and horses. Limited information is available about firocoxib in cattle, with only one study conducted in preweaned calves.[83] Pharmacokinetic parameters for firocoxib are presented in **Table 1**. Unique pharmacokinetic properties in preweaned calves include high oral bioavailability, prolonged terminal half-life, and an extensive tissue distribution (high volume of distribution).

Dehorning
An RCT to evaluate firocoxib was conducted on 4- to 6-week-old calves administered oral firocoxib (0.5 mg/kg) in combination with a lidocaine cornual nerve block administered 10 minutes before cautery dehorning.[84] Although the acute effects of cautery dehorning as determined by physiologic and nociception changes were unaffected by treatment, firocoxib-treated calves had an overall reduced integrated cortisol response in comparison with placebo-treated controls.

SEDATIVE-ANALGESIC DRUGS

The most commonly used sedative-analgesic drugs in veterinary practice are opioids, α2-agonists, and NMDA-receptor antagonists. When combined in doses considered too small to produce an effect alone, these compounds may act synergistically to produce an amplified effect. This effect is evident when combining subtherapeutic doses of xylazine (0.02–0.05 mg/kg), ketamine (0.05–0.1 mg/kg), and an opioid (butorphanol [0.05 mg/kg] or morphine [0.05 mg/kg]), which produces enhanced sedation in comparison with using these drugs individually.[85] This combination of sedatives is known as the "ketamine stun." Administration of these drugs may achieve rapid sedation and analgesia for improved animal welfare, handling, and reduced operator risk while conducting a painful procedure.

Opioid Analgesics

Opioids bind to the spinal and supraspinal receptors mu (μ), kappa (κ), and delta (δ), eliciting an analgesic effect.[86] Although all 3 receptors produce analgesia and an increased appetite, the μ receptor is primarily responsible for the observed adverse effects including respiratory depression, gastrointestinal hypomotility, nausea, sedation, and euphoria.[86]

As such, partial or mixed opioids may provide potent analgesia with reduced side effects. The US Drug Enforcement Agency (DEA) regulates narcotics and they are not approved for use in cattle in the United States; although their use would be permitted under AMDUCA following the requirements of ELDU.[86]

Butorphanol

Butorphanol is one of the more frequently used opioids in veterinary medicine. As a partial/mixed opioid, κ agonist, and either a partial μ agonist or antagonist, butorphanol continues to provide analgesia with the potential for fewer adverse effects compared with a complete μ agonist such as morphine.[86] Butorphanol is well tolerated, but its effects are limited to mild and moderate pain. Pharmacokinetic properties are presented in **Table 1**. The efficacy of butorphanol has not been investigated as an individual analgesic but rather in combination therapy (see later discussion).

Nalbuphine

Nalbuphine is an opioid that is a κ-receptor agonist and a μ-receptor antagonist. Similar to butorphanol, because of its mixed receptor activity, analgesia is induced with a decreased risk of adverse effects associated with a μ-receptor agonist.[86] Moreover, owing to the antagonism of the μ receptor, which is primarily responsible for dependency, the potential for abuse in humans is limited. Therefore, it is not considered a controlled schedule drug (except in Kentucky) because of the exclusion described in 21 C.F.R. § 1308.12 contained within the Controlled Substances Act (21 U.S.C. § 812).[87] This classification reduces storage and record-keeping responsibilities mandated for narcotics. The pharmacokinetics are listed in **Table 1**. The analgesic potency is noted to be similar to that of morphine, with pharmacologic effects similar to those of butorphanol.[86]

Castration

The efficacy of intravenous nalbuphine (0.4 mg/kg) administered immediately before surgical castration was investigated in an RCT.[88] Nalbuphine concentrations were rapidly eliminated, with no detectable concentrations 3 hours after the procedure. Although behaviors associated with acute pain were reduced in comparison with placebo-treated control calves, the investigators concluded that at the study dose, nalbuphine was unable to mitigate the physiologic stress of surgical castration for the study duration of 10 hours.[88]

α2-Adrenergic Agonists

α2-Adrenergic agonists produce a dose-dependent analgesic effect by inhibiting the amplification of norepinephrine (NE) release from the presynaptic nerve in the brainstem and spinal cord.[25,89] Analgesia is achieved through this reduction of NE, thereby inhibiting the afferent pain pathway.[89] Adverse effects can include decreased cardiac output, a centrally mediated decreased respiratory rate, and depressed gastrointestinal motility. These side effects can be reduced while maintaining analgesia through epidural administration. Although there is a longer onset for an epidural using xylazine rather than lidocaine (X: 12 $\pm$ 1 minutes vs L: 5 $\pm$ 1 minutes), duration is much improved (X: 303 $\pm$ 11 minutes vs L: 82 $\pm$ 12 minutes).[90] Combining these products provides the best of both properties, with a faster onset and prolonged duration (onset: 5 $\pm$ 1 minutes; duration: 253 $\pm$ 19 minutes).[90] Canadian veterinarians were more likely to use xylazine (>50%) than lidocaine (<30%) as a pain reliever when providing analgesia for castration.[91] Pharmacokinetics of xylazine are detailed in **Table 1**. Given its common use in cattle, previous studies have evaluated its potential as an analgesic.

Castration
Xylazine is associated with a reduced peak cortisol concentrations compared with castrated control calves.[32,46,92] This response is independent of route of administration (eg, epidural, intravenous)[32,92] or administration in combination with another analgesic compound, including flunixin.[46] However, the integrated cortisol response was equal to or greater than that in untreated control calves (see **Fig. 1**).[92] This finding is most likely due to the rebound in cortisol concentrations in xylazine-treated calves that occurs following the loss of analgesic activity. As such, xylazine should be used in combination with other analgesics that reduce the delayed inflammatory pain.

Dehorning
The response of xylazine administered perioperatively to calves being dehorned is similar to that for castration.[93] Compared with dehorned controls, the acute peak cortisol response is reduced in calves treated with intravenous xylazine (0.1 mg/kg); however, this effect does not persist past 3 hours.[93] With the addition of lidocaine to calves, the cortisol peak was further mitigated, but still the same cortisol profile was observed over time.[93] By contrast, Stilwell and colleagues[94] reported no difference in cortisol concentrations in calves treated with intramuscular xylazine (0.2 mg/kg) for the first hour after disbudding compared with saline-treated controls. Similarly to castration, the use of xylazine alone should be avoided for the development of analgesic protocols for dehorning.

Lameness
Administration of xylazine in combination with regional anesthesia immediately before claw surgery in cattle diagnosed with a sole ulcer resulted in pain relief in the acute stages when compared with placebo-treated controls; however, these effects were transient (<1 hour).[95]

N-Methyl-D-Aspartate Receptor Antagonists

Ketamine is a dissociative anesthetic commonly used in veterinary medicine. NMDA-receptor antagonists dampen brain activity by inhibiting the release of glutamate, an excitatory neurotransmitter.[96] Moreover, analgesia may also be produced through μ and κ opioid receptor binding, which occurs for both ketamine and its active metabolite, norketamine.[96] The analgesic potency of norketamine has been reported in a rat as one-third that of ketamine.[97] Pharmacokinetic parameters are reported in **Table 1**. Although NMDA-receptor antagonists are DEA-regulated,[87] given their analgesic and anesthesia properties and common use in veterinary medicine, studies have investigated their analgesic potential in combination with additional sedative-analgesics at subtherapeutic concentrations.

Combination Sedative-Analgesia Therapy

The combination of intravenous xylazine (0.05 mg/kg) and ketamine (0.1 mg/kg) reduced the peak cortisol in 4- to 6-month-old surgically castrated calves in comparison with placebo-treated castrated controls; however, the cortisol AUEC was greater in calves treated with xylazine and ketamine.[92] These results are most likely due to a rebound effect following the loss of drug activity. The short-lived effects of combination sedative-analgesia therapy are further supported by a study evaluating simultaneous castration and dehorning on 2- to 4-month-old dairy calves treated with subtherapeutic doses of butorphanol (0.025 mg/kg), xylazine (0.05 mg/kg), and ketamine (0.1 mg/kg).[67] Compared with placebo-treated calves, in castrated calves receiving the sedative combination for the first hour, cortisol concentrations were reduced; however, no significant differences were reported thereafter.[67] These combination sedative-analgesia therapies may find utility in a multimodal approach but appear to be ineffective when administered independently.

NEUROPATHIC PAIN ANALGESIC
Gabapentin

Gabapentin is a γ-aminobutyric acid (GABA) analogue historically used as an antiseizure medication. In addition, improved management of chronic, neuropathic pain has been reported, likely due to a decreased excitatory neurotransmitter release as a result of modulation of voltage-gated calcium channels.[98] Furthermore, analgesic activity can be enhanced with the addition of an NSAID because of a reported synergism.[99,100] Pharmacokinetic properties are listed in **Table 1**. As control of chronic pain is challenging, gabapentin has been investigated to address this concern.

Dehorning

Gabapentin (15 mg/kg), alone or in combination with meloxicam (1 mg/kg), has demonstrated an increased ADG in 6-month-old cattle following scoop dehorning; however, additional physiologic responses were no different from those in placebo-treated controls.[50]

Lameness

Following induction of a lameness model using amphotericin B, 4- to 6-month-old calves were treated with gabapentin (15 mg/kg) with or without meloxicam (0.5 mg/kg) once daily for 4 days.[21] Although gabapentin alone tended to demonstrate a beneficial response compared with placebo-treated controls, analgesia was most evident in the group receiving combination therapy, demonstrated by an increased stride length and force applied to the ipsilateral claw.[21]

SUMMARY

As managing pain in cattle remains challenging, several compounds have been investigated in RCTs to support their inclusion in the development of analgesia protocols. Evidence suggests that the use of local anesthetics, NSAIDs, opioids, α2-agonists, NMDA-receptor antagonists, and gabapentin may provide pain relief. Furthermore, combinations of these drug classes using a multimodal approach will optimize pain management in cattle. The use of meloxicam, ketoprofen, and flunixin in analgesic protocols, especially when combined with a local anesthetic, is supported by the results of RCTs. Sedative-analgesics do not provide prolonged pain relief as a singular treatment, and therefore should be used in combination with other analgesic classes. The AMDUCA regulates the extralabel use of analgesics in cattle within the United States.

ACKNOWLEDGMENTS

The authors acknowledge the assistance of Mal Hoover at Kansas State University in preparing the article for publication.

REFERENCES

1. Muir WW 3rd, Woolf CJ. Mechanisms of pain and their therapeutic implications. J Am Vet Med Assoc 2001;219:1346–56.
2. Gottschalk A, Smith DS. New concepts in acute pain therapy: preemptive analgesia. Am Fam Physician 2001;63:1979–84.
3. Kissin I. Preemptive analgesia. Anesthesiology 2000;93:1138–43.
4. Ochroch EA, Mardini IA, Gottschalk A. What is the role of NSAIDs in pre-emptive analgesia? Drugs 2003;63:2709–23.
5. Stafford KJ, Mellor DJ. The welfare significance of the castration of cattle: a review. N Z Vet J 2005;53:271–8.
6. Stafford KJ, Mellor DJ. Dehorning and disbudding distress and its alleviation in calves. Vet J 2005;169:337–49.
7. Coetzee JF. A review of analgesic compounds used in food animals in the United States. Vet Clin North Am Food Anim Pract 2013;29:11–28.
8. Stafford KJ, Mellor DJ. Addressing the pain associated with disbudding and dehorning in cattle. Appl Anim Behav Sci 2011;135:226–31.
9. Heinrich A, Duffield TF, Lissemore KD, et al. The effect of meloxicam on behavior and pain sensitivity of dairy calves following cautery dehorning with a local anesthetic. J Dairy Sci 2010;93:2450–7.
10. Ballou MA, Sutherland MA, Brooks TA, et al. Administration of anesthetic and analgesic prevent the suppression of many leukocyte responses following surgical castration and physical dehorning. Vet Immunol Immunopathol 2013; 151:285–93.
11. Sutherland MA, Ballou MA, Davis BL, et al. Effect of castration and dehorning singularly or combined on the behavior and physiology of Holstein calves. J Anim Sci 2013;91:935–42.
12. Mosher RA, Wang C, Allen PS, et al. Comparative effects of castration and dehorning in series or concurrent castration and dehorning procedures on stress responses and production in Holstein calves. J Anim Sci 2013;91:4133–45.
13. Woolf CJ, Mannion RJ. Neuropathic pain: aetiology, symptoms, mechanisms, and management. Lancet 1999;353:1959–64.
14. Smith GW, Davis JL, Tell LA, et al. FARAD digest - Extralabel use of nonsteroidal anti-inflammatory drugs in cattle. J Am Vet Med Assoc 2008;232:697–701.
15. Animal Medicinal Drug Use Clarification Act of 1994 (AMDUCA). U.S. Food and Drug Administration website. Available at: http://www.fda.gov/AnimalVeterinary/GuidanceComplianceEnforcement/ActsRulesRegulations/ucm085377.htm. Accessed October 10, 2014.
16. Coetzee JF. A review of pain assessment techniques and pharmacological approaches to pain relief after bovine castration: practical implications for cattle production within the United States. Appl Anim Behav Sci 2011;192–213.
17. Stock ML, Baldridge SL, Griffin D, et al. Bovine dehorning: assessing pain and providing analgesic management. Vet Clin North Am Food Anim Pract 2013;29:103–33.
18. Whay HR, Webster AJ, Waterman-Pearson AE. Role of ketoprofen in the modulation of hyperalgesia associated with lameness in dairy cattle. Vet Rec 2005; 157:729–33.

19. Flower FC, Sedlbauer M, Carter E, et al. Analgesics improve the gait of lame dairy cattle. J Dairy Sci 2008;91:3010–4.

20. Chapinal N, de Passille AM, Rushen J, et al. Effect of analgesia during hoof trimming on gait, weight distribution, and activity of dairy cattle. J Dairy Sci 2010;93: 3039–46.

21. Coetzee JF, Mosher RA, Anderson DE, et al. Impact of oral meloxicam administered alone or in combination with gabapentin on experimentally induced lameness in beef calves. J Anim Sci 2014;92:816–29.

22. Wong CH, Jenne CN, Lee WY, et al. Functional innervation of hepatic iNKT cells is immunosuppressive following stroke. Science 2011;334:101–5.

23. Coetzee JF, Edwards LN, Mosher RA, et al. Effect of oral meloxicam on health and performance of beef steers relative to bulls castrated on arrival at the feedlot. J Anim Sci 2012;90:1026–39.

24. Coetzee JF. Assessment and management of pain associated with castration in cattle. Vet Clin North Am Food Anim Pract 2013;29:75–101.

25. Webb AI, Pablo LS. Injectable anaesthetic agents. In: Riviere JE, Papich MG, editors. Veterinary pharmacology and therapeutics. 9th edition. Ames (IA): Wiley-Blackwell; 2009. p. 381–99.

26. Catterall WA, Mackie K. Local anesthetics. In: Brunton LL, Chabner BA, Knollmann BC, editors. Goodman & Gilman's manual of pharmacology and therapeutics. 12th edition. New York: McGraw-Hill Medical; 2011. p. 565–82.

27. Fierheller EE, Caulkett NA, Haley DB, et al. Onset, duration and efficacy of four methods of local anesthesia of the horn bud in calves. Vet Anaesth Analg 2012; 39:431–5.

28. Lomax S, Windsor PA. Topical anesthesia mitigates the pain of castration in beef calves. J Anim Sci 2013;91:4945–52.

29. Muir WW, Hubbell JA, Skarda R, et al. Local anesthesia in cattle, sheep, goats, and pigs. In: Muir WM, Hubbell JA, Skarda R, et al, editors. Handbook of veterinary anesthesia. 2nd edition. St Louis (MO): Mosby; 1995. p. 53–77.

30. Webster HB, Morin D, Jarrell V, et al. Effects of local anesthesia and flunixin meglumine on the acute cortisol response, behavior, and performance of young dairy calves undergoing surgical castration. J Dairy Sci 2013;96: 6285–300.

31. Earley B, Crowe MA. Effects of ketoprofen alone or in combination with local anesthesia during the castration of bull calves on plasma cortisol, immunological, and inflammatory responses. J Anim Sci 2002;80:1044–52.

32. Ting ST, Earley B, Hughes JM, et al. Effect of ketoprofen, lidocaine local anesthesia, and combined xylazine and lidocaine caudal epidural anesthesia during castration of beef cattle on stress responses, immunity, growth, and behavior. J Anim Sci 2003;81:1281–93.

33. Ting ST, Earley B, Crowe MA. Effect of repeated ketoprofen administration during surgical castration of bulls on cortisol, immunological function, feed intake, growth, and behavior. J Anim Sci 2003;81:1253–64.

34. Sorkin LS, Wallace MS. Acute pain mechanisms. Surg Clin North Am 1999;79: 213–29.

35. Stewart M, Stookey JM, Stafford KJ, et al. Effects of local anesthetic and a nonsteroidal antiinflammatory drug on pain responses of dairy calves to hot-iron dehorning. J Dairy Sci 2009;92:1512–9.

36. Grondahl-Nielsen C, Simonsen HB, Lund JD, et al. Behavioural, endocrine and cardiac responses in young calves undergoing dehorning without and with use of sedation and analgesia. Vet J 1999;158:14–20.

37. Doherty TJ, Kattesh HG, Adcock RJ, et al. Effects of a concentrated lidocaine solution on the acute phase stress response to dehorning in dairy calves. J Dairy Sci 2007;90:4232–9.
38. Morisse JP, Cotte JP, Huonnic D. Effect of dehorning on behavior and plasma cortisol response in young calves. Appl Anim Behav Sci 1995;43:239–47.
39. Shearer JK, Stock ML, Van Amstel SR, et al. Assessment and management of pain associated with lameness in cattle. Vet Clin North Am Food Anim Pract 2013;29:135–56.
40. Grosser T, Smyth E, FitzGerald GA. Anti-inflammatory, antipyretic, and analgesic agents: pharmacotherapy of gout. In: Brunton LL, Chabner BA, Knollmann BC, editors. Goodman & Gilman's manual of pharmacology and therapeutics. 12th edition. New York: McGraw-Hill Medical; 2011. p. 959–1004.
41. Svensson CI, Yaksh TL. The spinal phospholipase-cyclooxygenase-prostanoid cascade in nociceptive processing. Annu Rev Pharmacol Toxicol 2002;42: 553–83.
42. Lees P. Analgesics, antiinflammatory, antipyretic drugs. In: Riviere JE, Papich MG, editors. Veterinary pharmacology and therapeutics. 9th edition. Ames (IA): Wiley-Blackwell; 2009. p. 457–92.
43. Rubio F, Seawall S, Pocelinko R, et al. Metabolism of carprofen, a nonsteroid anti-inflammatory agent, in rats, dogs, and humans. J Pharm Sci 1980;69: 1245–53.
44. Stilwell G, Lima MS, Broom DM. Effects of nonsteroidal anti-inflammatory drugs on long-term pain in calves castrated by use of an external clamping technique following epidural anesthesia. Am J Vet Res 2008;69:744–50.
45. Currah JM, Hendrick SH, Stookey JM. The behavioral assessment and alleviation of pain associated with castration in beef calves treated with flunixin meglumine and caudal lidocaine epidural anesthesia with epinephrine. Can Vet J 2009;50:375–82.
46. Gonzalez LA, Schwartzkopf-Genswein KS, Caulkett NA, et al. Pain mitigation after band castration of beef calves and its effects on performance, behavior, Escherichia coli, and salivary cortisol. J Anim Sci 2010;88:802–10.
47. Stilwell G, de Carvalho RC, Lima MS, et al. Effect of caustic paste disbudding, using local anaesthesia with and without analgesia, on behaviour and cortisol of calves. Appl Anim Behav Sci 2009;35–44.
48. Huber J, Arnholdt T, Mostl E, et al. Pain management with flunixin meglumine at dehorning of calves. J Dairy Sci 2013;96:132–40.
49. Fraccaro E, Coetzee JF, Odore R, et al. A study to compare circulating flunixin, meloxicam and gabapentin concentrations with prostaglandin E(2) levels in calves undergoing dehorning. Res Vet Sci 2013;95:204–11.
50. Glynn HD, Coetzee JF, Edwards-Callaway LN, et al. The pharmacokinetics and effects of meloxicam, gabapentin, and flunixin in postweaning dairy calves following dehorning with local anesthesia. J Vet Pharmacol Ther 2013;36:550–61.
51. Stilwell G, Lima MS, Broom DM. Comparing plasma cortisol and behaviour of calves dehorned with caustic paste after non-steroidal-anti-inflammatory analgesia. Livest Sci 2008;119:63–9.
52. Allen KA, Coetzee JF, Edwards-Callaway LN, et al. The effect of timing of oral meloxicam administration on physiological responses in calves after cautery dehorning with local anesthesia. J Dairy Sci 2013;96:5194–205.
53. Schulz KL, Anderson DE, Coetzee JF, et al. Effect of flunixin meglumine on the amelioration of lameness in dairy steers with amphotericin B-induced transient synovitis-arthritis. Am J Vet Res 2011;72:1431–8.

54. Veterinary Medicine Expert Committee on Drug Information, USP. USP veterinary pharmaceutical information monographs—anti-inflammatories. J Vet Pharmacol Ther 2004;27(Suppl 1):1–110.

55. Aberg G, Ciofalo VB, Pendleton RG, et al. Inversion of (R)- to (S)-ketoprofen in eight animal species. Chirality 1995;7:383–7.

56. Stafford KJ, Mellor DJ, Todd SE, et al. Effects of local anaesthesia or local anaesthesia plus a non-steroidal anti-inflammatory drug on the acute cortisol response of calves to five different methods of castration. Res Vet Sci 2002; 73:61–70.

57. McMeekan CM, Stafford KJ, Mellor DJ, et al. Effects of regional analgesia and/or a non-steroidal anti-inflammatory analgesic on the acute cortisol response to dehorning in calves. Res Vet Sci 1998;64:147–50.

58. Sutherland MA, Mellow DJ, Stafford KJ, et al. Cortisol responses to dehorning of calves given a 5-h local anaesthetic regimen plus phenylbutazone, ketoprofen, or adrenocorticotropic hormone prior to dehorning. Res Vet Sci 2002;73: 115–23.

59. Milligan BN, Duffield T, Lissemore K. The utility of ketoprofen for alleviating pain following dehorning in young dairy calves. Can Vet J 2004;45:140–3.

60. Duffield TF, Heinrich A, Millman ST, et al. Reduction in pain response by combined use of local lidocaine anesthesia and systemic ketoprofen in dairy calves dehorned by heat cauterization. Can Vet J 2010;51:283–8.

61. Faulkner PM, Weary DM. Reducing pain after dehorning in dairy calves. J Dairy Sci 2000;83:2037–41.

62. Chapinal N, de Passille AM, Rushen J, et al. Automated methods for detecting lameness and measuring analgesia in dairy cattle. J Dairy Sci 2010;93:2007–13.

63. Newby NC, Pearl DL, LeBlanc SJ, et al. The effect of administering ketoprofen on the physiology and behavior of dairy cows following surgery to correct a left displaced abomasum. J Dairy Sci 2013;96:1511–20.

64. Smith G. Extralabel use of anesthetic and analgesic compounds in cattle. Vet Clin North Am Food Anim Pract 2013;29:29–45.

65. Coetzee JF, Gehring R, Bettenhausen AC, et al. Attenuation of acute plasma cortisol response in calves following intravenous sodium salicylate administration prior to castration. J Vet Pharmacol Ther 2007;30:305–13.

66. Gingerich DA, Baggot JD, Yeary RA. Pharmacokinetics and dosage of aspirin in cattle. J Am Vet Med Assoc 1975;167:945–8.

67. Baldridge SL, Coetzee JE, Dritz SS, et al. Pharmacokinetics and physiologic effects of intramuscularly administered xylazine hydrochloride-ketamine hydrochloride-butorphanol tartrate alone or in combination with orally administered sodium salicylate on biomarkers of pain in Holstein calves following castration and dehorning. Am J Vet Res 2011;72:1305–17.

68. Kotschwar JL, Coetzee JF, Anderson DE, et al. Analgesic efficacy of sodium salicylate in an amphotericin B-induced bovine synovitis-arthritis model. J Dairy Sci 2009;92:3731–43.

69. Delatour P, Foot R, Foster AP, et al. Pharmacodynamics and chiral pharmacokinetics of carprofen in calves. Br Vet J 1996;152:183–98.

70. Strub KM, Aeppli L, Muller RK. Pharmacological properties of carprofen. Eur J Rheumatol Inflamm 1982;5:478–87.

71. Pang WY, Earley B, Sweeney T, et al. Effect of carprofen administration during banding or Burdizzo castration of bulls on plasma cortisol, in vitro interferon-gamma production, acute-phase proteins, feed intake, and growth. J Anim Sci 2006;84:351–9.

72. Pang WY, Earley B, Murray M, et al. Banding or Burdizzo castration and carprofen administration on peripheral leukocyte inflammatory cytokine transcripts. Res Vet Sci 2011;90:127–32.
73. Stilwell G, Lima MS, Carvalho RC, et al. Effects of hot-iron disbudding, using regional anaesthesia with and without carprofen, on cortisol and behaviour of calves. Res Vet Sci 2012;92:338–41.
74. Stock ML, Barth LB, Van Engen, et al. Impact of carprofen administration on the stress and nociception response in cautery dehorned calves [abstract]. World Buiatrics Congress XXVII. Cairns, Australia, July 27–August 1, 2014.
75. Coetzee JF, KuKanich B, Mosher R, et al. Pharmacokinetics of intravenous and oral meloxicam in ruminant calves. Vet Ther 2009;10:E1–8.
76. Repenning PE, Ahola JK, Callan RJ, et al. Impact of oral meloxicam administration before and after band castration on feedlot performance and behavioral response in weanling beef bulls. J Anim Sci 2013;91:4965–74.
77. Heinrich A, Duffield TF, Lissemore KD, et al. The impact of meloxicam on postsurgical stress associated with cautery dehorning. J Dairy Sci 2009;92:540–7.
78. Coetzee JF, Mosher RA, KuKanich B, et al. Pharmacokinetics and effect of intravenous meloxicam in weaned Holstein calves following scoop dehorning without local anesthesia. BMC Vet Res 2012;8:153.
79. Theurer ME, White BJ, Coetzee JF, et al. Assessment of behavioral changes associated with oral meloxicam administration at time of dehorning in calves using a remote triangulation device and accelerometers. BMC Vet Res 2012;8:48.
80. Offinger J, Herdtweck S, Rizk A, et al. Postoperative analgesic efficacy of meloxicam in lame dairy cows undergoing resection of the distal interphalangeal joint. J Dairy Sci 2013;96:866–76.
81. Newby NC, Tucker CB, Pearl DL, et al. Short communication: a comparison of 2 nonsteroidal antiinflammatory drugs following the first stage of a 2-stage fistulation surgery in dry dairy cows. J Dairy Sci 2013;96:6514–9.
82. Fitzpatrick CE, Chapinal N, Petersson-Wolfe CS, et al. The effect of meloxicam on pain sensitivity, rumination time, and clinical signs in dairy cows with endotoxin-induced clinical mastitis. J Dairy Sci 2013;96:2847–56.
83. Stock ML, Gehring R, Barth LA, et al. Pharmacokinetics of firocoxib in preweaned calves after oral and intravenous administration. J Vet Pharmacol Ther 2014;37:457–63.
84. Stock ML, Gehring R, Millman ST, et al. Attenuation of the integrated cortisol response following administration of oral firocoxib in preweaned calves prior to cautery disbudding [abstract]. 2014 ADSA-ASAS-CSAS Joint Annual Meeting. Kansas City (MO), July 20–24, 2014.
85. Abrahamsen EJ. Chemical restraint, anesthesia, and analgesia for camelids. Vet Clin North Am Food Anim Pract 2009;25:455–94.
86. Kukanich B, Papich MG. Opioid analgesic drugs. In: Riviere JE, Papich MG, editors. Veterinary pharmacology and therapeutics. 9th edition. Ames (IA): Wiley-Blackwell; 2009. p. 301–35.
87. DEA. Drug scheduling. U.S. Drug Enforcement Administration. Available at: http://www.justice.gov/dea/pubs/scheduling.html. Accessed October 17, 2014.
88. Coetzee JF, Lechtenberg KF, Stock ML, et al. Pharmacokinetics and effect of intravenous nalbuphine in weaned Holstein calves after surgical castration. J Vet Pharmacol Ther 2014;37:169–77.
89. Adams HR. Adrenergic agonists and antagonists. In: Riviere JE, Papich MG, editors. Veterinary pharmacology and therapeutics. 9th edition. Ames (IA): Wiley-Blackwell; 2009. p. 125–55.

90. Grubb TL, Riebold TW, Crisman RO, et al. Comparison of lidocaine, xylazine, and lidocaine-xylazine for caudal epidural analgesia in cattle. Vet Anaesth Analg 2002;29:64–8.

91. Hewson CJ, Dohoo IR, Lemke KA, et al. Canadian veterinarians' use of analgesics in cattle, pigs, and horses in 2004 and 2005. Can Vet J 2007;48:155–64.

92. Coetzee JF, Gehring R, Tarus-Sang J, et al. Effect of sub-anesthetic xylazine and ketamine ('ketamine stun') administered to calves immediately prior to castration. Vet Anaesth Analg 2010;37:566–78.

93. Stafford KJ, Mellor DJ, Todd SE, et al. The effect of different combinations of lignocaine, ketoprofen, xylazine and tolazoline on the acute cortisol response to dehorning in calves. N Z Vet J 2003;51:219–26.

94. Stilwell G, Carvalho RC, Carolino N, et al. Effect of hot-iron disbudding on behaviour and plasma cortisol of calves sedated with xylazine. Res Vet Sci 2010;88:188–93.

95. Rizk A, Herdtweck S, Offinger J, et al. The use of xylazine hydrochloride in an analgesic protocol for claw treatment of lame dairy cows in lateral recumbency on a surgical tipping table. Vet J 2012;192:193–8.

96. Annetta MG, Iemma D, Garisto C, et al. Ketamine: new indications for an old drug. Curr Drug Targets 2005;6:789–94.

97. Leung LY, Baillie TA. Comparative pharmacology in the rat of ketamine and its 2 principal metabolites, norketamine and (Z)-6-hydroxynorketamine. J Med Chem 1986;29:2396–9.

98. Taylor CP. Mechanisms of analgesia by gabapentin and pregabalin - Calcium channel alpha(2)-delta [Ca-v alpha(2)-delta] ligands. Pain 2009;142:13–6.

99. Hurley RW, Chatterjea D, Feng MH, et al. Gabapentin and pregabalin can interact synergistically with naproxen to produce antihyperalgesia. Anesthesiology 2002;97:1263–73.

100. Picazo A, Castaneda-Hernandez G, Ortiz MI. Examination of the interaction between peripheral diclofenac and gabapentin on the 5% formalin test in rats. Life Sci 2006;79:2283–7.

Evidence for the Use of Ceftiofur for Treatment of Metritis in Dairy Cattle

Emily J. Reppert, DVM, MS

KEYWORDS

• Dairy cattle • Metritis • Uterine disease • Ceftiofur • Cephalosporin

KEY POINTS

• Uterine disease, such as metritis, is frequently diagnosed in postpartum dairy cattle.
• The treatment of puerperal metritis includes the use of antibiotics.
• Evidence supports the use of ceftiofur for the treatment of metritis.

INTRODUCTION

Uterine disease, such as metritis, is common in postpartum dairy cows. Metritis is capable of affecting a large number of animals in a herd and is associated with production losses.[1,2] Microbial infections of the reproductive tract can result in infertility by disrupting normal uterine and ovarian function. The incidence of uterine disease within the first week postpartum has been documented to be as high as 40%.[3] Herd incidence of metritis largely depends on the definition of disease. Several large surveys have identified ranges of clinical metritis and puerperal metritis to be between 36% and 50%[4,5] and 18% and 21%,[6,7] respectively. Despite being an important production disease in dairy cattle, clinical metritis and puerperal metritis have only been recently defined. The lack of a uniform clinical definition has made interpretation of current research, treatment, and prognosis challenging. In 2006, Sheldon and colleagues[8] proposed definitions for clinical and puerperal metritis to provide guidelines for treatment and prognosis. Both clinical and puerperal metritis are characterized by an enlarged uterus with fetid red-brown uterine discharge within the first 21 days in milk.[8] The definition distinguishes clinical and puerperal metritis by the presence of a fever and systemic involvement in the latter. Histologically, metritis is characterized by inflammation of all layers of the uterine wall with edema, infiltration of leukocytes, and degeneration of the myometrium.

The author does not have anything to disclose.
Veterinary Health Center, Kansas State University, 1800 Denison Avenue, Manhattan, KS 66506, USA
E-mail address: emilyjeanreppert@gmail.com

Vet Clin Food Anim 31 (2015) 139–149
http://dx.doi.org/10.1016/j.cvfa.2014.11.007   **vetfood.theclinics.com**

Inflammation of the uterine mucosa is associated with leukocyte infiltration secondary to uterine infection with *Escherichia coli*, *Trueperella pyogenes*, and *Fusobacterium necrophorum*.[9–11] The severity of disease associated with puerperal metritis warrants treatment with supportive care and antibiotics. Antibiotic treatments for metritis have included penicillin and ceftiofur.[8,12,13] In 2012, the Food and Drug Administration (FDA) issued a final rule prohibiting certain extralabel uses of cephalosporins in food animals.[14] This ruling limits the extralabel use of cephalosporins in food animals to only those cephalosporins with an approved regimen in that species, and use for any purpose in food animals must conform to the label regimen, with the exception of the first-generation cephalosporin, cephapirin. At the time of this publication, only ceftiofur hydrochloride (Excenel RTU-EZ; Zoetis, Madison, NJ) and ceftiofur crystalline-free acid (Excede Sterile Suspension; Zoetis) are labeled for the treatment of bovine metritis in the United States. This article analyzes the available evidence for the use of ceftiofur for the treatment of metritis in postpartum dairy cattle.

PATIENT EVALUATION

Metritis is found in dairy cattle within the first 21 days in milk and most commonly within the first 7 days postpartum. The severity of the disease and distinction between puerperal and clinical metritis is associated with the presence or absence of systemic illness. In 2006 Sheldon and colleagues[8] proposed the following definitions to aide in diagnosis and classification of puerperal and clinical metritis:

- Puerperal metritis: enlarged uterus with a fetid watery red-brown uterine discharge, associated with systemic signs of illness including decreased milk production, depression, anorexia, and other signs of toxemia and fever greater than 39.5°C (103.1°F), within 21 days postpartum
- Clinical metritis: enlarged uterus and purulent uterine discharge within 21 days after parturition

Abnormalities in rectal temperature and evaluation of vaginal discharge have been the mainstay for clinical diagnosis of puerperal and clinical metritis. However, it is important that rectal temperature and vaginal discharge be interpreted together because there is evidence that a portion of healthy postpartum dairy cows have an elevated rectal temperature within the first 10 days in milk.[15]

Risk factors for the development of metritis include retained fetal membranes, dystocia, twins, stillbirth, and ketosis.[16–18] A large field study performed by Markusfeld[4] provided evidence that primiparous cows may be at greater risk for development of metritis when compared with multiparous cows. Rapid and accurate diagnosis of metritis is necessary to allow for initiation of appropriate treatment, detection of severity of disease, and prognostication for future fertility of the animal.

PHARMACOLOGIC TREATMENT OPTIONS
Antibiotic Therapy

Animals affected by puerperal metritis have moderate to severe systemic disease and should be treated. The basis of treatment has been antibiotics and supportive care. The focus of treatment in this article was the administration of systemic antibiotics for the treatment of puerperal metritis, hereafter referred to as metritis. The drug chosen to treat metritis should be effective against those pathogens isolated from the infected uterus. The most common bacteria associated with metritis include *E coli*, *T pyogenes*, and a range of anaerobes including *Prevotella* species and *F necrophorum*.[19–21] The diverse group of organisms isolated from cows with metritis warrants the use of broad-spectrum antibiotics. Antibiotics that have been used to treat metritis include penicillin, oxytetracycline, ampicillin, and ceftiofur.[6,12] A large body of recent research has evaluated ceftiofur for the treatment of metritis. Ceftiofur has been found to reach therapeutic concentrations within all layers of the uterus and in lochia.[22] Administration of ceftiofur to cows with evidence of postpartum fever and uterine discharge showed significant improvement in cure rates, milk yield, and rectal temperature.[15] Although there is evidence to support the use of ceftiofur, the lack of a uniform clinical definition and the diversity in types and dosages of ceftiofur used has made interpretation of current research difficult. This article uses an evidence-based approach to summarize the current evidence for the use of ceftiofur as the treatment of metritis.

Materials and Methods

To establish the efficacy of ceftiofur against metritis in dairy cattle a bibliographic search was performed using the online databases PubMed and CAB abstracts. The keywords "dairy cattle," "metritis," and "ceftiofur" were used for the search. Additional articles were found by an exhaustive review of the references from the articles found via the online databases.

Only controlled prospective experimental studies were evaluated. To be eligible for review, the articles had to meet additional criteria: diagnosis of metritis defined as a rectal temperature greater than or equal to 39.5°C (103.1°F) with fetid red-brown vaginal discharge occurring within the first 21 days in milk; treatment of metritis had to include a group of cows treated with ceftiofur alone; and outcome of treatment had to be objectively measured as a decrease in rectal temperature, change in milk production, improvement in the character of vaginal discharge, or alteration in reproductive performance. Eligible articles were further evaluated to determine the type of ceftiofur given, and the route and the dose of administration. The quality of each article was determined as described by Vandeweerd and colleagues[23] by being scored. The score was based on a set of criteria that each article needed to have within each portion of the paper. The maximum possible quality score was 100%. Article quality was arbitrarily categorized as high (>60%), intermediate (45%–60%), and low quality (<45%).

Results

Fig. 1 represents the article selection process. A total of 52 articles were identified using the search terms "dairy cattle," "metritis," and "ceftiofur." Initial screening of the titles of the 52 articles revealed 18 articles for further review. Of the 18 articles, 12 met the exclusion criteria for the paper leaving six articles for further analysis. The reasons for exclusion included lack of a treatment group where ceftiofur was used as the sole treatment (N = 4), absence of a definition for metritis or the definition did not comply with the inclusion criteria (N = 3), administration of ceftiofur was used as prophylaxis and not as treatment of metritis (N = 1), incomplete data (N = 2), language other than English (N = 1), and experimental induction of metritis rather than naturally occurring disease (N = 1).

Table 1 summarizes general information about the six papers[6,12,13,24–26] that were included in the analysis. The six articles used for this study were written in English. Of the six articles, five[6,13,25–27] were considered high quality (scores 86, 68, 70, 88, 74) and one[12] was considered intermediate quality (score 51). Three[13,25,27] of the six articles had untreated negative control groups and three[6,12,26] had treated positive control groups.

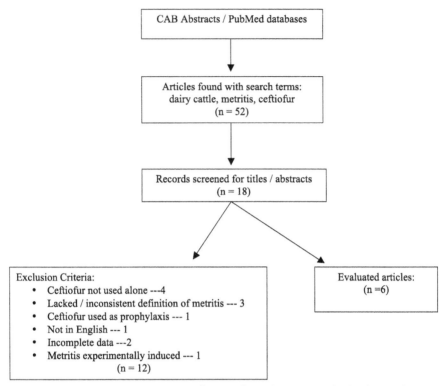

Fig. 1. Flow chart for systematic review of the evidence for the use of ceftiofur for the treatment of metritis in dairy cattle.

The six experimental studies tested the efficacy of ceftiofur for the treatment of metritis. Metritis was defined as an elevated rectal temperature (>39.5°C [103.1°F] in four articles[6,13,26,27] and >39.2°C [102.6°F] in two articles[12,25]) with fetid red-brown vaginal discharge occurring within the first 21 days in milk. Efficacy of ceftiofur was measured by clinical cure in the six articles. The clinical cure as a response to treatment was defined as a decrease in rectal temperature alone[6,12,13]; a combination of a decrease in rectal temperature and absence of fetid vaginal discharge[13,25,26]; or a decrease in rectal temperature, an absence of fetid vaginal discharge, and no additional antibiotic therapy needed.[27] Other parameters evaluated included reproductive performance,[6,25,26] milk production,[12,24] endometritis,[25] acute-phase proteins,[12] and financial analysis.[6]

Treatment Efficiency

Table 2 summarizes the results from each of the selected studies. In the six articles, three different ceftiofur antibiotics were evaluated: (1) ceftiofur hydrochloride (Excenel RTU, Pfizer Animal Health, New York, NY[13]; Excenel, Pharmacia and Upjohn, Erlangen, Germany[6]; Ceobiotic, Tecnofarm SRL, Buenos Aires, Argentina[25]; Excenel RTU, Zoetis[25]), (2) ceftiofur crystalline-free acid (Pfizer Animal Health Inc[26], Kalamazoo, MI), and (3) ceftiofur sodium Naxcel (The Upjohn Co[12]). Efficacy of ceftiofur was determined by clinical cure in all six studies. Two[13,26] of the negative control studies, representing the pivotal efficacy studies for ceftiofur hydrochloride and

Table 1
Summary of articles

Year	Country	Study Population	Control Group	# of Animals	Ceftiofur	Route	Dose	Study Strength
2004	United States	Holstein	Negative control	406	CHCL	SC and IM	1.1 mg/kg 2.2 mg/kg IM or SC for 5 d	Strong
2001	Germany	German Black Pied	Positive control[a]	325	CHCL	IM	600 mg	Strong
2013	Argentina	Holstein	Negative control	284	CHCL	IM	2.2 mg/kg	Strong
2014	United States	Not specified	Positive control[b]	528	CHCL	IM	2.2 mg/kg	Strong
2012	United States	Holstein	Negative control	1023	CCFA	SC	6.6 mg/kg twice, 2 d apart	Strong
1998	United States	Holstein	Positive control[c]	51	CNA	IM	2.2 mg/kg IM for 5 d	Intermediate

Abbreviations: CCFA, ceftiofur crystalline-free acid; CHCL, ceftiofur hydrochloride; CNA, ceftiofur sodium; IM, intramuscular; SC, subcutaneous.

[a] Positive control animals consisted of two groups: (1) intrauterine pills containing 2500 mg ampicillin and 2500 mg cloxacillin, in addition to 6000 mg ampicillin IM; (2) same intrauterine pill regimen as other treatment but with 500 mg ceftiofur IM on 3 consecutive days.

[b] Positive control animals consisted of 1 mg/kg ampicillin trihydrate once daily for 5 days.

[c] Positive control animals consisted of two groups: (1) 22,000 IU/kg procaine penicillin G IM for 5 days; (2) same penicillin G regimen plus intrauterine infusion of 6 g of oxytetracycline on Days 1, 3, and 5.

Data from Refs.[6,12,13,24–26]

Table 2
Summary of the results of treatment with ceftiofur

Ceftiofur	Time of Treatment	Results – Clinical Cure	Duration of Treatment
CHCL	1–14 dpp	Significant reduction in rectal temperature compared with control animals ($P \leq .012$ at both doses during treatment period) Clinical cure rates significantly greater for treated animals ($P = .01$ at a dose of 2.2 mg/kg)	5 d
CHCL	4–6 dpp	Significant decrease in rectal temperature in all groups No significant difference between treatments on cure rate	3 d
CHCL	4–5 dpp	No significant differences in fever between treatment groups	3–5 d
CHCL	5–7 dpp	No significant effect on cure at 21 DIM ($P > .01$)	3 d
CHCL	1–12 dpp	Clinical cure more rapid for ampicillin-treated animals Animals with puerperal metritis had decreased clinical cure compared with animals with clinical metritis	5 d
CCFA	1–10 dpp	Clinical cure greater for ceftiofur-treated animals ($P < .0001$) Significant effect of ceftiofur on rectal temperature compared with control animals on Days 1, 5, and 6 of study ($P \leq .0003$)	2 doses 72 h apart
CCFA	1–4 dpp 5–10 dpp	No significant differences in cure rates among treatment groups	1 dose on day of diagnosis
CNA	3–10 dpp	No significant difference in temperature reduction among treatment groups	5 d

Abbreviations: CCFA, ceftiofur crystalline-free acid; CHCL, ceftiofur hydrochloride; CNA, ceftiofur sodium; DIM, days in milk; dpp, days postpartum.
Data from Refs.[6,12,13,24–28]

ceftiofur crystalline-free acid, showed that ceftiofur treatment significantly improved clinical cure. The other negative control study[25] did not demonstrate a treatment effect of ceftiofur hydrochloride. Three[6,12,25] studies did not detect a significant effect of ceftiofur on clinical cure as compared with positive control groups, including ampicillin tridydrate (Polyflex; Boehringer Ingelheim Vetmedica, St. Joseph, MO), and combinations of penicillin or ampicillin and uterine boluses.

Of the studies that evaluated the effect of ceftiofur on reproductive performance of cows diagnosed with metritis, two[6,25] found no statistical difference when the ceftiofur treatments were compared with positive control animals; one study found that the risk of pregnancy in animals treated with ceftiofur was greater than the negative control group.[24] The papers that evaluated milk production as a response to treatment found that ceftiofur-treated animals had a numerical increase in milk production but there was no significant difference from the positive or negative control groups.[12,24] The study investigating the effect of ceftiofur on the development of endometritis found that treatment of metritis with ceftiofur did not have a significant effect on the number of animals that went on to develop endometritis as compared with negative control animals.[24] However, Lima and colleagues[25] found a difference in the development of endometritis at 32 days in milk between cows that had been treated with ampicillin and those treated with ceftiofur. The cows that had fetid vaginal discharge and were treated with ceftiofur had a greater prevalence of purulent vaginal discharge (endometritis) at 32 days in milk compared with cows that had been treated with ampicillin. Acute-phase proteins were measured in study and overall there was an increase in acute-phase proteins in animals diagnosed with metritis compared with control animals but there was no significant effect of treatment with ceftiofur versus positive control animals of either procaine penicillin G alone, or combined with intrauterine infusion of oxytetracycline.[12]

DISCUSSION

Metritis results from inflammation of all layers of the uterus within the first 7 days postpartum. Predisposing factors for disease include retained fetal membranes, dystocia, and metabolic derangements.[16–18] The definition of puerperal metritis was most recently defined as uterine inflammation resulting in systemic signs of illness, including fever, red-brown watery fetid uterine discharge, dullness, anorexia, elevated heart rate, and decreased production.[8] The systemic nature and sometimes serious side effects of the disease warrant treatment with antibiotics. Systemic antibiotics that have been used include penicillin, oxytetracycline, ampicillin, and ceftiofur.[6,12] Ceftiofur has been specifically evaluated as a treatment of postpartum inflammation and has been shown to reach therapeutic concentrations in the uterus and in lochia.[22] The effect of ceftiofur on postpartum inflammation and fever has also been assessed and it was found that systemic administration significantly improved cure rate, milk yield, and rectal temperature in postpartum dairy cows with fever and vaginal discharge or dystocia.[15] This article critically evaluates the evidence for treatment of metritis with ceftiofur. The primary criteria for inclusion in the review was based on the current definition of metritis by Sheldon and colleagues[8] and all studies had to use ceftiofur for the treatment of clinical metritis. Maintaining a strict definition for inclusion may have eliminated some studies that provide strong evidence for the use of ceftiofur, such as the study by Zhou and colleagues.[15]

A semiobjective method of ranking the quality of the studies was performed based on the recent article by Vandeweerd and colleagues.[23] Each article was evaluated and given a score out of 100. The ranking was based on a list of questions provided in the article. Ideally, more than one reviewer would have performed the ranking. In this review, the author ranked only the articles that could serve as a potential source of bias. Nonetheless, the ranking process for the selected articles revealed strong evidence for the use of ceftiofur for the treatment of metritis. However, it was difficult to evaluate the efficacy of ceftiofur among the studies because they varied by the definition of clinical cure, the type of ceftiofur used, the doses, and the lack of a negative control group in several of the papers.

The lack of a consistent definition of clinical cure made it difficult to compare the efficacy of ceftiofur among the studies. Most papers considered the combination of a decrease in rectal temperature and/or improvement in the character of vaginal discharge in the definition of cure. However, the studies varied as to when treatments were initiated, when rectal temperature was first measured, and when clinical cure was assessed. Consistency in timing of treatment and diagnosis may be important especially in those studies evaluating a decrease in rectal temperature as clinical cure. In 2007, a study by Benzaquen and colleagues[7] evaluated the diagnoses of puerperal metritis and rectal temperature and found that a portion of cows became febrile before being diagnosed with puerperal metritis. Such findings may suggest that treatment early in the course of disease may alter the development of a fever associated with puerperal metritis. However, interpretation of pyrexia in the postpartum period needs to be taken in context with other clinical signs, because there is evidence that postpartum pyrexia is not consistently associated with bacterial contamination of the uterus.[27]

Another challenge in determining the effect of ceftiofur on the treatment of metritis was the inconsistency in control groups. All studies evaluated in the review had a control group. To determine efficacy of ceftiofur, there needed to be a group of animals with metritis that remained as untreated control subjects. However, only three of the studies had negative control groups that consisted of cows diagnosed with metritis.[13,24,26] The other studies[6,12,25] had positive control groups made up of animals that had recently calved and were healthy. The studies[6,12,25] that did not have a negative control group compared ceftiofur with another drug that was an accepted method of treatment of metritis. The conclusion that can be made from those studies, in the presence of statistical significance with proper statistical analysis, is that one of the antimicrobials resulted in a different clinical response rate than the other. Lack of significant differences in positive control studies cannot automatically be considered as proof of equivalence of the test articles, the most important reason being that of the potential for insufficient statistical power to give the illusion of product equivalence. Noninferiority studies require specific design considerations, including the outcome difference that would be considered as equivalent, and consideration of the variance likely to be encountered in the outcomes. The FDA Center for Veterinary Medicine Guidance for Industry #204 documents the components of an appropriate noninferiority study.[28] To evaluate the efficacy of ceftiofur alone, future studies should include negative control groups.

In 2012, the FDA restricted the extralabel use of third-generation cephalosporins in certain food-producing animals in the United States. The regulations specifically prohibit extralabel doses and extralabel routes of administration of the antibiotic in major food-producing species, such as cattle.[14] At the time of this publication there were two ceftiofur products with label indications for the treatment of metritis in the United States. Of the studies reviewed in this article only three[13,25,26] of the papers administered ceftiofur at the labeled dose and route of administration currently approved by the FDA.[14] In light of the new ceftiofur regulations, finding alternative antibiotics for the treatment of metritis may be warranted. The study by Lima and coworkers[25] provided some evidence that cows treated with ampicillin resulted in a more rapid clinical cure compared with cows treated with ceftiofur making ampicillin a potential alternative treatment. However, this study lacked a negative control group.

Of the studies evaluated in this review, two large field trials by Chenault and colleagues[13] and McLaughlin and colleagues[26] provide the strongest evidence for the use of ceftiofur for the treatment of metritis in dairy cattle. In each paper the clinical cure was clearly defined, there was a large sample size, and there was a negative control group. Chenault and colleagues[13] evaluated two different doses of ceftiofur hydrochloride (1.1 mg/kg vs 2.2 mg/kg) and found a statistically significant decrease in rectal temperature between cows treated with the higher dose of ceftiofur and control animals. McLaughlin and colleagues[26] found similar results in cows treated with two doses (6.6 mg/kg) of ceftiofur crystalline-free acid administered 72 hours apart having a statistically significant decrease in rectal temperature compared with untreated control animals. Additionally, both studies used ceftiofur according to label indications and would be considered legal in the United States.

The body of literature evaluating the efficacy of antibiotics other than ceftiofur for the treatment of metritis is limited. In the preparation of this article, an additional literature review was performed to identify all papers analyzing the efficacy of oxytetracycline for the treatment of metritis. The search identified 34 articles. Of the articles, only six were prospective[12,29–33] and only three had a group of cows treated with oxytetracycline alone.[12,29,30] Analysis and interpretation of treatment effect was made further difficult because of the lack of negative control animals, inconsistent definition of metritis, and variation in the dose and the route of administration of the drug. The review supports the need for further prospective negative controlled studies with clear definitions of disease for the evaluation of the efficacy of all antibiotics for the treatment of metritis.

SUMMARY

This article evaluates evidence for the use of ceftiofur for the treatment of metritis in dairy cattle. Based on a semiobjective analysis there were eight well-designed articles evaluating the use of ceftiofur. The lack of negative control groups and small samples sizes for some of the studies may limit their usefulness in determining the effect of ceftiofur alone. Future research should include larger studies with negative control groups.

REFERENCES

1. Fourichon C, Seegers H, Bareille N, et al. Effects of disease on milk production in the dairy cow: a review. Prev Vet Med 1999;41(1):1–35.
2. Fourichon C, Seegers H, Malher X. Effect of disease on reproduction in the dairy cow: a meta-analysis. Theriogenology 2000;53(9):1729–59.
3. Sheldon IM, Cronin J, Goetze L, et al. Defining postpartum uterine disease and the mechanisms of infection and immunity in the female reproductive tract in cattle. Biol Reprod 2009;81(6):1025–32.
4. Markusfeld O. Periparturient traits in seven high dairy herds. Incidence rates, association with parity, and interrelationships among traits. J Dairy Sci 1987; 70(1):158–66.
5. Zwald NR, Weigel KA, Chang YM, et al. Genetic selection for health traits using producer-recorded data. I. Incidence rates, heritability estimates, and sire breeding values. J Dairy Sci 2004;87(12):4287–94.
6. Drillich M, Beetz O, Pfützner A, et al. Evaluation of a systemic antibiotic treatment of toxic puerperal metritis in dairy cows. J Dairy Sci 2001;84(9):2010–7.
7. Benzaquen ME, Risco CA, Archbald LF, et al. Rectal temperature, calving-related factors, and the incidence of puerperal metritis in postpartum dairy cows. J Dairy Sci 2007;90(6):2804–14.
8. Sheldon IM, Lewis GS, Leblanc S, et al. Defining postpartum uterine disease in cattle. Theriogenology 2006;65(8):1516–30.
9. Miller AN, Williams EJ, Sibley K, et al. The effects of *Arcanobacterium pyogenes* on endometrial function in vitro, and on uterine and ovarian function in vivo. Theriogenology 2007;68(7):972–80.
10. Bicalho RC, Machado VS, Bicalho ML, et al. Molecular and epidemiological characterization of bovine intrauterine *Escherichia coli*. J Dairy Sci 2010;93(12): 5818–30.
11. Santos TM, Gilbert RO, Bicalho RC. Metagenomic analysis of the uterine bacterial microbiota in healthy and metritic postpartum dairy cows. J Dairy Sci 2011;94(1): 291–302.
12. Smith BI, Donovan GA, Risco C, et al. Comparison of various antibiotic treatments for cows diagnosed with toxic puerperal metritis. J Dairy Sci 1998;81(6):1555–62.

13. Chenault JR, Mcallister JF, Chester ST, et al. Efficacy of ceftiofur hydrochloride sterile suspension administered parenterally for the treatment of acute postpartum metritis in dairy cows. J Am Vet Med Assoc 2004;224(10):1634–9.

14. New Animal Drug; Cephalosporins Drugs; Extralabel Animal Drug Use; Order of Prohibition. Food and Drug Administration: Register The Daily Journal of the United States Government. Federal Register. 77;4 Friday, January 6, 2012. 733–44.

15. Zhou C, Boucher JF, Dame KJ, et al. Multilocation trial of ceftiofur for treatment of postpartum cows with fever. J Am Vet Med Assoc 2001;219(6):805–8.

16. Gröhn YT, Erb HN, Mcculloch CE, et al. Epidemiology of metabolic disorders in dairy cattle: association among host characteristics, disease, and production. J Dairy Sci 1989;72(7):1876–85.

17. Correa MT, Erb H, Scarlett J. Path analysis for seven postpartum disorders of Holstein cows. J Dairy Sci 1993;76(5):1305–12.

18. Suthar VS, Canelas-raposo J, Deniz A, et al. Prevalence of subclinical ketosis and relationships with postpartum diseases in European dairy cows. J Dairy Sci 2013; 96(5):2925–38.

19. Griffin JF, Hartigan PJ, Nunn WR. Non-specific uterine infection and bovine fertility. I. Infection patterns and endometritis during the first seven weeks postpartum. Theriogenology 1974;1(3):91–106.

20. Messier S, Higgins R, Couture Y, et al. Comparison of swabbing and biopsy for studying the flora of the bovine uterus. Can Vet J 1984;25(7):283–8.

21. Sheldon IM, Noakes DE, Rycroft AN, et al. Influence of uterine bacterial contamination after parturition on ovarian dominant follicle selection and follicle growth and function in cattle. Reproduction 2002;123(6):837–45.

22. Okker H, Schmitt EJ, Vos PL, et al. Pharmacokinetics of ceftiofur in plasma and uterine secretions and tissues after subcutaneous postpartum administration in lactating dairy cows. J Vet Pharmacol Ther 2002;25(1):33–8.

23. Vandeweerd JM, Clegg P, Hougardy V, et al. Using systematic reviews to critically appraise the scientific information for the bovine veterinarian. Vet Clin North Am Food Anim Pract 2012;28(1):13–21, vii.

24. Giuliodori MJ, Magnasco RP, Becu-villalobos D, et al. Metritis in dairy cows: risk factors and reproductive performance. J Dairy Sci 2013;96(6):3621–31.

25. Lima FS, Vieira-neto A, Vasconcellos GS, et al. Efficacy of ampicillin trihydrate or ceftiofur hydrochloride for treatment of metritis and subsequent fertility in dairy cows. J Dairy Sci 2014;97(9):5401–14.

26. Mclaughlin CL, Stanisiewski E, Lucas MJ, et al. Evaluation of two doses of ceftiofur crystalline free acid sterile suspension for treatment of metritis in lactating dairy cows. J Dairy Sci 2012;95(8):4363–71.

27. Sheldon IM, Rycroft AN, Zhou C. Association between postpartum pyrexia and uterine bacterial infection in dairy cattle. Vet Rec 2004;154(10):289–93.

28. Guidance for Industry. Active controls in studies to demonstrate effectiveness of a new animal drug for use in companion animals. Available at: http://www.fda.gov/downloads/AnimalVeterinary/GuidanceComplianceEnforcement/GuideforIndustry/UCM308680. Accessed October 22, 2014.

29. Bhat FA, Bhattacharyya HK. Management of metritis in crossbred cattle of Kashmir using oxytetracycline, cephalexin and prostaglandin F 2alpha. Indian J Anim Res 2012;46(2):187–9.

30. Bretzlaff KN, Whitmore HL, Spahr SL, et al. Incidence and treatments of postpartum reproductive problems in a dairy herd. Theriogenology 1982;17(5):527–35.

31. Dawson LJ, Aalseth EP, Hawman CH, et al. Reproductive performance of dairy cows after early detection and oxytetracycline treatment of post-partum metritis. Bov Pract 1988;23:24–8.
32. Liu W, Chuang S, Shyu C, et al. Strategy for the treatment of puerperal metritis and improvement of reproductive efficiency in cows with retained placenta. Acta Vet Hung 2011;59(2):247–56.
33. Nak Y, Dagalp SB, Cetin C, et al. Course and severity of postpartum metritis cases following antibiotic and PGF 2alpha administration in postpartum metritis cows infected with BoHV-4. Transbound Emerg Dis 2011;58(1):31–6.

Consideration of Evidence for Therapeutic Interventions in Bovine Polioencephalomalacia

 CrossMark

Michael D. Apley, DVM, PhD

KEYWORDS

- Polioencephalomalacia • Bovine • Thiamine • Dexamethasone • Furosemide
- Mannitol • Dimethyl sulfoxide • Nonsteroidal anti-inflammatory drugs

KEY POINTS

- Randomized, masked, prospective clinical trial evidence for therapeutic intervention in naturally occurring bovine polioencephalomalacia is nonexistent.
- Mechanistic, physiologic, and induced model data support the use of thiamine in the therapy of bovine polio.
- The use of nonsteroidal anti-inflammatory drugs and dexamethasone in the therapy of bovine polio are not supported by available induced model data and literature reviews of human data.
- Dimethyl sulfoxide has demonstrated efficacy against cerebral edema in induced models in laboratory animals, but lack of clinical trial confirmation in bovine polio and issues with legality of many of the available formulations call for caution in clinical use at this time.
- There are no clinical trial data to support the use of the diuretics furosemide or mannitol for bovine polioencephalomalacia; research data for mannitol demonstrate varying efficacy and potential adverse reactions depending on the mechanism of cerebral edema and status of the blood-brain barrier.

INTRODUCTION

In contrast to other articles in this issue, the volume of clinical outcome data for bovine polioencephalomalacia therapy borders on nonexistent. This article evaluates the use of thiamine and anti-inflammatories in the therapy of polioencephalomalacia based on available information related to the pathophysiology of the disease, induced models, disease outcome in other species (sheep), and parallels in similar disease in humans.

The author has nothing to disclose.
Department of Clinical Sciences, Kansas State University College of Veterinary Medicine, 1800 Denison Avenue, Manhattan, KS 66506, USA
E-mail address: mapley@vet.ksu.edu

POLIO PATHOPHYSIOLOGY

In 1956, Jensen and colleagues[1] described the neuropathology of widespread polio cases in cattle located in Colorado, Wyoming, western Kansas, and western Nebraska, mentioning a clinical similarity to blind staggers thought at that time to be associated with selenium toxicity. In 1969, Little and Sorenson described polio in feedlot cattle in Minnesota, referencing a relationship to thiamine deficiency, but recognizing the lack of clarity as to the cause of this deficiency in the face of adequate dietary thiamine.[2] By 1997, there were 13 articles demonstrating the association of excess sulfur in the ration and/or water with polio.[3]

In a 1998 review, Gould[4] pointed out that there is confusion in the literature as to how the term "polioencephalomalacia" is used. It can be used in reference to a softening of the gray matter of the brain (cerebrocortical necrosis), which may be attributed to altered thiamine status, water deprivation–sodium ion toxicosis, lead poisoning, or high sulfur intake. Polioencephalomalacia also may be used in reference to a neurologic disease syndrome associated with an altered thiamine status.

The reader is directed to Gould's review[4] for an in-depth discussion of the different etiologies of polio, but for the purposes of this article, it should be noted that the relationship of thiamine deficiency and polio is uncertain. In contrast, the association of sulfur-associated polio with excessive ruminal sulfide production has been demonstrated; more specifically, the production of abnormal quantities of hydrogen sulfide gas.[5] A review of thiamine status in the blood and sulfide in rumen fluid in steers with acute signs of polio as compared with normal steers revealed no alterations in thiamine status but significant alterations in ruminal sulfide concentrations during the time of highest polio occurrence at approximately 3 weeks on feed.[6]

In a 2013 publication, Amat and colleagues[7] conducted an induced model study and a field investigation of a field polio outbreak, along with an extensive literature review. In an induced polio model, these investigators evaluated rumen, blood, and brain concentrations of thiamine and the active metabolites thiamine monophosphate (TMP) and thiamine diphosphate (TDP). The 35-day study treatments consisted of a 2 × 2 factorial design incorporating low (0.3% dry matter) and high (0.67% dry matter) sulfur rations, and 2 differing concentrate-containing rations (4 heifers for each treatment combination). Thiamine was added to all diets at a low level, although the method of reporting in the article does not allow reporting of mg/kg body weight intake. No heifers displayed signs of polio during the study or histologic lesions of polio at necropsy. Results indicated that dietary sulfur had no effect on total thiamine and esters in the rumen fluid or blood. However, the heifers receiving high-sulfur ration had higher total thiamine concentrations in the brain compared with those on low-sulfur diets ($P<.01$), with a numerical decrease in free thiamine ($P = .35$) and numerical increase in TDP ($P = .10$).

Amat and colleagues[7] also reported on an outbreak of naturally occurring polio in feedlot heifers that occurred in close temporal proximity to the induced model study. Eighteen heifers were affected in the outbreak. The calculated total sulfur intake of the heifers in the natural outbreak was close to the high-sulfur intake group in the induced model; the feed was tested and found to contain 0.34% sulfur and the water contained 1755 ppm sulfate. Total sulfur intake from feed and water was estimated to be 47 g per head per day. Treatment consisted of 20 mg dexamethasone intravenously (IV) (Dexamethasone 5, 5 mg/mL; Vetquinol, Lavaltries, Quebec, Canada) and a combination of florfenicol and flunixin meglumine (Resflor, 6 mL/45 kg subcutaneously (SC); Merck Animal Health, Kirkland, Quebec, Canada), and later treated with trimethoprim-sulfamethazine and thiamine (Thiamine Hydrochloride Injection USP, 100 mg/mL thiamine hydrochloride, 2 mL/45 kg; Dominion Veterinary Laboratories, Ltd, Winnipeg, Manitoba, Canada). This thiamine regimen equates to approximately 4.4 mg/kg. The number of administrations of thiamine, time from diagnosis to treatment, or time from initial treatment to death of the 4 mortalities in the outbreak were not reported.

In comparing the normal brains in the induced model study with the brains of the 4 heifers that died or were euthanized in the clinical outbreak, the outbreak heifers had lower concentrations of total thiamine phosphates, with the TDP concentrations 36.5% lower than the experimental heifers. In contrast, the free thiamine concentrations were 4.9-fold higher than the normal brains in the experimental heifers.

This article advances the understanding of the relationship of sulfur and thiamine metabolism by proposing 2 main hypotheses for this interaction. The first is that clinical polio may be due to an inability to convert free thiamine to TDP in the brain, which leads to major deficits in energy metabolism. Thiamine diphosphate is synthesized by the action of pyrophosphokinase (TPK) on thiamine. This enzyme is based on adequate availability of the substrate (thiamine), ATP, and Mg^{2+}. From the work in both induced models and the clinical outbreak, it is apparent that the lack of the thiamine substrate is a poor hypothesis. However, the reported adverse effects of sulfite on ATP production in mitochondria and Mg^{2+} absorption from the rumen raise the need for future research in these interactions, as these actions could significantly decrease the activity of TPK. A second hypothesis from the authors is that the strong nucleophile characteristics of sulfite, and the fact that TDP is a very active molecule that is very susceptible to degradation by nucleophiles, raises the possibility that there is direct degradation of TDP by sulfites.

Bettendorf and colleagues noted in 1996 that while the functions of TMP and thiamine triphosphate (TTP) are not yet well described, TDP has been demonstrated to be a key component of several vital energy metabolism pathways.[8] Bettendorf and colleagues again reviewed the function of thiamine in polio in 2014;[9] in mammalian brains, free thiamine and TMP have no known physiologic function and account for 5% to 15% of total thiamine. TDP accounts for 80% to 90% of total thiamine and is a vital cofactor for pyruvate, oxoglutarate dehydrogenases, and transketolase. Only approximately 1% of thiamine present in the brain is composed of TTP and the recently discovered forms adenosine thiamine triphosphate and adenosine thiamine diphosphate; these 3 forms are thought to play an as-yet undetermined role in intracellular messaging and metabolic regulation.

The relationship of thiamine phosphorylated metabolites to neurologic function has been well documented in humans. Thiamine deficiency in humans is encountered when intake is insufficient due to malnutrition, such as with chronic alcoholism, gastrointestinal disease, and HIV-AIDS.[10] In these cases, Wernicke encephalopathy often results, a key characteristic of which is neuronal loss. Alcohol also has been shown to inhibit the formation of TDP. The neurodegenerative effects of Alzheimer and Parkinson diseases also have been linked to decreased activities of thiamine-dependent enzymes in the presence of adequate thiamine availability.

Hazell and Butterworth[11] reviewed cell damage mechanisms due to thiamine deficiency, finding that oxidative stress, excitotoxicity, and inflammation were primary outcomes. These results are informative to polio in cattle because of the similar lack of TDP in both cases. The review focused on the pathology of Wernicke encephalopathy. Oxidative stress and the production of nitric oxide have been demonstrated in thiamine deficiency models; nitric oxide has been correlated with decreased activity of α-ketoglutarate dehydrogenase. Oxidative stress also has been linked to break down of the blood-brain barrier, which has been demonstrated to occur in thiamine deficiency.

Hazell and Butterworth[11] also reviewed the literature on the effects of thiamine deficiency on the focal accumulation of lactic acid in the brain, which results in cyto-toxic edema. Vasogenic edema due to the breakdown of the blood-brain barrier also is a cause of the edema seen in Wernicke encephalopathy. Inflammation has been documented to be a major part of human neurologic diseases, such as stroke, multiple sclerosis, and Alzheimer disease; involvement of inflammation in the pathology of thiamine deficiency also is suggested by microglial reactivity and production of proinflammatory cytokines.

Whether the lack of TDP is due to primary thiamine deficiency or the lack of formation of TDP from adequately available thiamine, it is clear that the lack of TDP availability in the brain results in a wide-reaching cascade of pathologic events leading to neuronal cell death.

THERAPY AND PREVENTION OF POLIO WITH THIAMINE

Thiamine has been used as both a preventive and therapeutic treatment. It is available in North America as 200 and 500 mg/mL thiamine hydrochloride injectable products with multiple labels. It also is available as a powder for feed supplementation. In vitamin B complex injectable products, thiamine hydrochloride (vitamin B_1) is included at 12.5 mg/mL in standard products and at 100 mg/mL in "fortified" products. One product has thiamine hydrochloride included at 150 mg/mL. It is important to evaluate the label of the thiamine product being used because of a wide variety of concentrations.

The appropriate regimen for thiamine in the therapy of bovines would best be described as empirical. A dose of 10 to 20 mg/kg intramuscularly (IM) or SC every 8 hours for up to 3 days in the absence of clinical response has been recommended.[12] In severe cases, IV administration has been proposed, but the thiamine should be diluted and administered slowly in recognition of potential adverse reactions. These investigators suggest that polio resulting from molasses-urea intake may respond very poorly to thiamine.

Although thiamine has been proposed for inclusion in cattle rations at doses of 1 g per head per day, there is no evidence this dose is effective. Review of the doses used in studies cited later in this article would suggest that much higher doses would be necessary for any possible effect.

Clear guidance in the form of clinical trials in naturally occurring polio in cattle is not available. Therefore, it is necessary to evaluate induced disease models, clinical outcomes from similar diseases in other species, and physiologic indicators. Reports of thiamine used for therapy of polio in the literature consist only of case reports. Although these cannot be considered definitive proof of the effect of thiamine, they are informative as to the variety of situations in which sulfur-related polio may occur and the variety of thiamine therapeutic regimens used in the field.

In a 1965 letter to the editor of the *Veterinary Record*, Davies[13] cited reported responses to thiamine (regimen not reported) in cattle displaying clinical signs of what would be diagnosed as polio; he also requested other veterinarians to report their experiences with this therapy. One animal showed initial response to thiamine after being laterally recumbent for 24 hours; it was able to stand, then relapsed and improved again in response to thiamine therapy. Subsequent euthanasia and histologic examination demonstrated extensive necrosis of the cerebral cortex. The suggestion in the letter that therapy earlier in the disease may have been successful is consistent with observations of failure in polio therapy today. However, the discussion of the potential issues with thiamine metabolism related to sulfur suggests that regardless of thiamine regimen and timing, the formation of sufficient TDP to overcome the pathology of sulfur-induced polio may not be consistently remedied by providing more thiamine as substrate.

Beke and Hironaka[14] described polio occurring in 4 yearling heifers exposed to sulfur in saline well water. The only source of water contained 2250 mg/L (ppm) of sulfate. The heifers were treated once with 5000 mg thiamine IV and then this dose was repeated IM every 12 hours for 2 days. All 4 heifers recovered.

Jeffrey[15] reported on an outbreak of ammonium sulfate–induced polio in cattle and sheep on several farms in England. All of the farms had introduced a new ration containing ammonium sulfate instead of the normal urinary acidifier ammonium bicarbonate. The affected cases were treated with 5 to 10 mg/kg body weight of thiamine, some daily for 3 days. No cases were identified as responding to the therapy, and new cases ceased when the supplement was withdrawn. All necropsied cases had cerebrocortical necrosis and necrosis in the thalamus and/or the striatum.

Bulgin and colleagues[16] reported that 28 of 40 ewes, which had grazed alfalfa sprayed with elemental sulfur, survived after treatment with 2000 mg of thiamine IM and 1800 mg of a 200 mg/mL oxytetracycline product. Recovery occurred over a period of 30 days. These 40 ewes still displayed clinical signs the day after exposure, with 206 of 2200 yearling ewes dying before their treatment. Ten other ewes left with the flock developed clinical signs and died approximately 3 days after clinical signs became apparent. Necropsies confirmed polio in the mortalities associated with the exposure.

Sheep have been used as an experimental model for induction of polio and the effect of thiamine on lesion development. A study by Olkowski and colleagues[17] evaluated the effects of 0.19% and 0.63% sulfur diets in a 2 × 2 factorial study with either 14 or 243 mg thiamine per kg of diet for 14 weeks to lambs that were 2 months old at the start of the study. Seven of 22 lambs fed the high-sulfur diet with low thiamine supplementation developed polio between the third and eighth weeks of the study. All of these animals had lesions in their cortex, midbrain, and brainstem that were consistent with polio. In addition, several of the lambs without clinical symptoms had brain lesions at necropsy. None of the lambs from the other groups developed clinical symptoms. The investigators postulated that thiamine inadequacy leading to polio in the face of excess sulfur may be the result of an increased thiamine requirement.

In a rat model of alcoholism, thiamine supplementation also has been shown to contribute to more rapid recovery of hepatic and neuronal damage when alcohol was discontinued after 90 days of administration at 4 g alcohol per kilogram body weight.[18] During the period immediately following cessation of alcohol administration, the levels of markers of fibrosis and inflammation reversed more quickly over 30 days when the rats received 25 mg thiamine/100 g body weight (250 mg/kg) orally, daily, as compared with just cessation of alcohol administration alone. In this case, the antioxidant properties of thiamine were credited with assisting in the reversal of oxidative stress–induced alcohol damage.

ANTI-INFLAMMATORY THERAPY OF POLIO

The author has noted veterinarians using ancillary therapy for polio consisting of dexamethasone, dimethyl sulfoxide (DMSO), or flunixin meglumine. Dexamethasone, DMSO, and furosemide have been mentioned in the literature as being used to address cerebral edema encountered in polio.[19] A textbook reference suggests a single IV dose of sodium dexamethasone at 0.1 to 0.2 mg/kg, or 1 g/kg of mannitol in a 20% solution administered IV may be beneficial in reducing cerebral edema.[12]

Literature searches using PubMed, CAB, and Agricola failed to locate clinical trials in bovine polio with any of these compounds. Therefore, without clinical trials in naturally occurring disease, therapeutic decisions must be informed by induced models, physiologic indicators, and trial information in other species.

In reviewing evidence from studies of cerebral edema and neuronal cell necrosis from other causes than polio, it is important to recognize that differences in pathophysiology may lead to differing results than if these drugs were applied in bovine polio. However, in absence of clear guidance, looking for trends in available research is a reasonable approach to inform therapeutic decisions.

Nonsteroidal Anti-inflammatory Therapy

There is evidence that inhibition of the prostaglandin production in neurologic disease is not uniformly beneficial. Gu and colleagues[20] evaluated a highly specific cyclooxygenase 2 (COX-2) inhibitor, nimesulide, in a thiamine-deficiency rat model, which results in neuronal cell death in vulnerable areas of the rat brain. The pathology is attributed to depletion of TDP stores that subsequently decrease the activity of α-ketoglutarate dehydrogenase, in turn limiting the rate of activity of the tricarboxylic acid cycle. The resulting mitochondrial dysfunction leads to neuronal cell death. The model showed that COX-2 activity in vulnerable areas of the brain was increased 200% with a resulting increase in prostaglandin E_2 (PGE_2) production of 200% to 300%. Administration of nimesulide resulted in significantly reduced PGE_2 concentrations in the vulnerable areas, which was associated with exacerbated neuronal cell death. The investigators cited the literature to establish the wide variation in the results of using COX-2 inhibitors in neurodegenerative diseases, varying from beneficial to adverse effects on treatment outcome.

Lleo and colleagues,[21] in an extensive review of nonsteroidal anti-inflammatory drugs (NSAIDs) in neurodegenerative diseases of humans, stated that the notion must be dispelled that brain inflammation encompasses a stereotypical set of all-purpose reactions, and that complexity arises in relation to stage of disease development and the type of disease. The reviews by both Gu and colleagues[20] and Lleo and colleagues[21] support the concept that simply targeting inflammation, edema, or free radicals in bovine polio with NSAIDs without clinical trial confirmation of efficacy is not consistently supported by the physiologic evidence, and there is potential for both beneficial and detrimental effects.

Dexamethasone

Literature on dexamethasone therapy of neuronal disease suggests the need for caution in including dexamethasone in the therapy of central nervous diseases of cattle. A 1976 study by de la Torre and Surgeon[22] evaluated dexamethasone and DMSO in an experimental model of cerebral infarction in Rhesus monkeys. In their study, it was demonstrated that reduction in cerebral edema due to dexamethasone was not associated with improved neurologic status. The investigators reported on extensive literature as of the time of the study that showed equivocal results of dexamethasone used in treating cerebral edema as a major component of the pathologic sequelae following stroke.

Based on the hypothesis that alleviating vasogenic edema after status epilepticus would be neuroprotective, Duffy and colleagues[23] used MRI to evaluate the neuroprotective effect of dexamethasone in a lithium-pilocarpine–induced status epilepticus rat model. In this study, both 2 mg/kg and 10 mg/kg of dexamethasone sodium phosphate administered after cessation of status epilepticus were found to exacerbate the acute cerebral edema and brain injury.

Yang and colleagues[24] evaluated the effects of dexamethasone injected immediately after and 3 days after collagenase-induced intracerebral hemorrhage in rats. Their results demonstrate that this dexamethasone administration schedule reduced poststroke brain edema; however, through interpretation of this study and extensive literature, the investigators also recognized that the timing of administration may be critical. They cited dexamethasone benefits as including inhibition of oxygen free radical–induced lipid peroxidation, suppression of vasogenic edema, and inflammatory responses to brain edema. The investigators also stated that dexamethasone therapeutic results in intracerebral hemorrhage (ICH) are conflicting and that little is known about optimal timing of intervention. Diuretics and hyperosmolar therapy are the only proven methods of reducing edema and intracranial pressure in patients with ICH. Several references were cited to support the statement that the use of dexamethasone in nononcologic brain edema in humans is not just debatable, it is considered contraindicated and ineffective; however, dexamethasone remains as the primary drug for treatment of high-altitude cerebral edema.[25]

In the case of dexamethasone, the potential immunosuppression in cattle also must be evaluated. Roth and Kaeberle[26] used dexamethasone as a research model to suppress neutrophil function in cattle. A dose of 0.04 mg/kg daily (0.9 mL/100 lb of a 2 mg/mL solution) for 3 days was effective as a research model to suppress neutrophil function in cattle, allowing the evaluation of compounds to reverse this suppression. Chiang and colleagues[27] used this same regimen beginning 24 hours after initiating an induced *Histophilus somni* model to demonstrate that the dexamethasone-treated calves had increased extent and severity of pneumonic lesions 7 days after model initiation, and the only mortalities before study completion were from the dexamethasone group. Although the effects of a single dose are not necessarily evident from these studies, it is clear that cattle are very sensitive to the immunosuppressive effects of dexamethasone, and this potential must be considered any time this drug is administered to cattle.

It is recognized that the mechanisms of cerebral edema in bovine polio versus ICH, infarction, status epilepticus, and other neurodegenerative diseases of humans may be quite different. However, the wide variety of effects of dexamethasone in these cases and research models suggests caution in applying overly simplistic reasoning to support the use of dexamethasone in treatment of bovine polio, and perhaps other bovine central nervous system (CNS) diseases, such as thromboembolic meningoencephalitis and listeriosis.

Dimethyl Sulfoxide

DMSO lacks clinical trial confirmation for efficacy in therapy of bovine polio. Physiologic justification has included discussion of free radical scavenging and diuresis, but even induced model data for these benefits in polio are lacking. However, there are extensive reports of benefits of DMSO in the therapy of human CNS disease.

The study by de la Torre and Surgeon,[22] cited previously, demonstrated that DMSO was protective against ischemic damage in an induced cerebral infarction model. An extensive review of the use of DMSO in human CNS disease by Jacob and de la Torre[28] cited both model and clinical trial evidence for benefits of DMSO in the therapy of traumatic brain injury, spinal cord injury, and human stroke. Possible properties of DMSO leading to these effects were cited as suppression of cytotoxicity caused by excess glutamate release, restriction of toxic Na^+ and Ca^{2+} entry in cells, blockade of thrombosis caused by tissue factors, and reduction of intracranial pressure. An earlier review of the DMSO literature also outlined multiple properties and effects of

DMSO,[29] suggesting a possible application for some of the pathology encountered in bovine polio.

Although the intention is not to promote DMSO as a wonder drug for bovine polio, there is certainly physiologic evidence to encourage clinical investigation of efficacy. In clinical practice, the use of DMSO in cattle would need to be narrowly limited to products with a veterinary or human label under the Animal Medicinal Drug Use Clarification Act (AMDUCA) regulations.[30] Only one liquid DMSO product is evident in the list of approved veterinary products in a Food and Drug Administration Center for Veterinary Medicine Database (DOMOSO Solution, NADA Number: 032–168, Zoetis, Kalamazoo, MI).[31] In the case of a DMSO product meeting AMDUCA regulation requirements, the veterinarian would need to seek out information to allow assignment of an exaggerated withdrawal time. The Grade "A" Pasteurized Milk Ordinance allows no use or storage of nonmedical-grade DMSO in dairies.[32] Introduction of a solvent-grade DMSO, which does not have human or veterinary approval, into a food animal results in that animal being adulterated and unable to enter the food chain.

DIURETICS: MANNITOL AND FUROSEMIDE

The comparative ability of mannitol and furosemide to affect brain water has been compared in multiple studies in humans and laboratory animals. A study in human patients with primary and metastatic brain tumors used IV furosemide or IV mannitol to evaluate changes in brain density with computed tomography.[33] Although the mannitol induced an increase in brain density correlated with cerebral diuresis, no changes were observed after furosemide treatment despite induction of maximal systemic diuresis.

A study of mannitol and furosemide in normal rat brain found that mannitol was effective in reducing brain water content.[34] Citing the use of mannitol and furosemide to reduce increased intracranial pressure and brain bulk during neurosurgery, Thenuwara and colleagues[34] investigated this effect on anesthetized rats with normal brains. Mannitol produced a dose-dependent reduction in brain water content. Furosemide alone did not affect plasma osmolality or brain water at any of 3 doses; however, it was synergistic with mannitol in decreasing brain water. In an extensive review of the literature concerning furosemide and cerebral edema, the investigators noted that furosemide can alter intracellular water regulation in brain cells and that multiple investigators have reported that furosemide can decrease intracranial pressure in the face of no change in brain water content.

In a subsequent study, Todd and colleagues[35] evaluated the effect of mannitol and furosemide alone and in combination in rats subjected to fluid percussion injury of the left cerebral hemisphere. The experimental model induced increased water content in the affected hemisphere as compared with the contralateral hemisphere. Mannitol was effective in increasing plasma osmolality and reducing water content of both hemispheres, whereas furosemide produced no effect either alone or in combination with mannitol.

The use of mannitol to treat cerebral edema in humans was reviewed by Diringer and Zazulia in 2004.[36] Mannitol was cited as crossing neither the cell membrane nor the intact blood-brain barrier, with additional activity in inhibiting programmed cell death and as a free radical scavenger. However, mannitol is capable of crossing a damaged blood-brain barrier, with concerns about increasing cerebral edema in damaged areas of the brain and shifting fluid to these damaged areas from undamaged regions. Although mannitol has been proven effective in traumatic brain injury, the data for use in cerebral infarction of humans is less consistent; although most experimental models have demonstrated reduction in infarct size, edema, and neurologic deficit, 2 retrospective studies in humans found that mannitol was not effective in improving the neurologic condition of patients.[37,38] A prospective study of mannitol in patients with stroke found no benefit or harm.[38]

The literature suggests that furosemide would be ineffective in addressing cerebral edema associated with bovine polio. Although mannitol has been shown to be effective in improving clinical status of human patients in some forms of cerebral insults, therapeutic outcomes in other diseases are lacking clinical support of efficacy. The uncertain status of the blood-brain barrier in bovine polio cases, and lack of clear physiologic guidance in this disease, makes the use of mannitol equivocal with the potential for harm in the absence of guidance from clinical trials.

SUMMARY

The use of thiamine in the therapy of bovine polio is supported by data from induced models and other species, but primary clinical trial data are not available. Ancillary agents, such as NSAIDs, dexamethasone, DMSO, furosemide, and mannitol, have been used, but clinical trial confirmation is not available and other available data suggest varying potential for enhancing therapeutic outcome. In light of lack of substantial supportive data, the potential for each of these drugs to cause harm must be carefully considered before empiric inclusion in a treatment regimen for bovine polio.

REFERENCES

1. Jensen R, Griner LA, Adams OR. Polioencephalomalacia of cattle and sheep. J Am Vet Med Assoc 1956;129(7):311–21.
2. Little PB, Sorensen DK. Bovine polioencephalomalacia, infectious embolic meningoencephalitis, and acute lead poisoning in feedlot cattle. J Am Vet Med Assoc 1969;155(12):1892–903.
3. Olkowski AA. Neurotoxicity and secondary metabolic problems associated with low to moderate levels of exposure to excess dietary sulphur in ruminants: a review. Vet Hum Toxicol 1997;39(6):355–60.
4. Gould DH. Polioencephalomalacia. J Anim Sci 1998;76(1):309–14.
5. Loneragan GH, Gould DH, Callan RJ, et al. Association of excess sulfur intake and an increase in hydrogen sulfide concentrations in the ruminal gas cap of recently weaned beef calves with polioencephalomalacia. J Am Vet Med Assoc 1998;213(11):1599–604, 1571.
6. McAllister MM, Gould DH, Raisbeck MF, et al. Evaluation of ruminal sulfide concentrations and seasonal outbreaks of polioencephalomalacia in beef cattle in a feedlot. J Am Vet Med Assoc 1997;211(10):1275–9.
7. Amat S, McKinnon JJ, Olkowski AA, et al. Understanding the role of sulfur-thiamine interaction in the pathogenesis of sulfur-induced polioencephalomalacia in beef cattle. Res Vet Sci 2013;95(3):1081–7.
8. Bettendorff L, Mastrogiacomo F, Kish SJ, et al. Thiamine, thiamine phosphates, and their metabolizing enzymes in human brain. J Neurochem 1996;66(1):250–8.
9. Bettendorff L, Lakaye B, Kohn G, et al. Thiamine triphosphate: a ubiquitous molecule in search of a physiological role. Metab Brain Dis 2014.
10. Butterworth RF. Thiamin deficiency and brain disorders. Nutr Res Rev 2003;16(2):277–84.
11. Hazell AS, Butterworth RF. Update of cell damage mechanisms in thiamine deficiency: focus on oxidative stress, excitotoxicity and inflammation. Alcohol Alcohol 2009;44(2):141–7.

12. Cebra C, Loneragan GH, Gould DH. Polioencephalomalacia (cerebrocortical necrosis). In: Smith BP, editor. Large animal internal medicine. 5th edition. St Louis (MO): Elsevier; 2015. p. 954–6.
13. Davies ET. Cerebrocortical necrosis in calves. Vet Rec 1965;77(10):290.
14. Beke GJ, Hironaka G. Toxicity to beef cattle of sulfur in saline well water: a case study. Sci Total Environ 1991;101:281–90.
15. Jeffrey M. Polioencephalomalacia associated with the ingestion of ammonium sulphate by sheep and cattle. Vet Rec 1994;134(14):343–8.
16. Bulgin MS, Lincoln SD, Mather G. Elemental sulfur toxicosisi in a flock of sheep. J Am Vet Med Assoc 1996;208(7):1063–5.
17. Olkowski AA, Gooneratne SR, Rousseaux CG, et al. Role of thiamine status in sulphur induced polioencephalomalacia in sheep. Res Vet Sci 1992;52(1):78–85.
18. Vidhya A, Renjugopal V, Indira M. Impact of thiamine supplementation in the reversal of ethanol induced toxicity in rats. Indian J Physiol Pharmacol 2013;57(4):406–17.
19. Linnabary RD, Baldwin EW, Silva-Krott IU. Bovine polioencephalomalacia (PEM) with long-term clinical recovery. Agri Pract 1990;11(5):21–4.
20. Gu B, Desjardins P, Butterworth RF. Selective increase of neuronal cyclooxygenase-2 (COX-2) expression in vulnerable brain regions of rats with experimental Wernicke's encephalopathy: effect of nimesulide. Metab Brain Dis 2008;23(2):175–87.
21. Lleo A, Galea E, Sastre M. Molecular targets of non-steroidal anti-inflammatory drugs in neurodegenerative diseases. Cellular and molecular life sciences. Cell Mol Life Sci 2007;64(11):1403–18.
22. de la Torre JC, Surgeon JW. Dexamethasone and DMSO in experimental trans-orbital cerebral infarction. Stroke 1976;7(6):577–83.
23. Duffy BA, Chun KP, Ma D, et al. Dexamethasone exacerbates cerebral edema and brain injury following lithium-pilocarpine induced status epilepticus. Neurobiol Dis 2014;63:229–36.
24. Yang JT, Lee TH, Lee IN, et al. Dexamethasone inhibits ICAM-1 and MMP-9 expression and reduces brain edema in intracerebral hemorrhagic rats. Acta Neurochir (Wien) 2011;153(11):2197–203.
25. Luks AM, Swenson ER. Medication and dosage considerations in the prophylaxis and treatment of high-altitude illness. Chest 2008;133(3):744–55.
26. Roth JA, Kaeberle ML. In vivo effect of ascorbic acid on neutrophil function in healthy and dexamethasone-treated cattle. Am J Vet Res 1985;46(12):2434–6.
27. Chiang YW, Roth JA, Andrews JJ. Influence of recombinant bovine interferon gamma and dexamethasone on pneumonia attributable to *Haemophilus somnus* in calves. Am J Vet Res 1990;51(5):759–62.
28. Jacob SW, de la Torre JC. Pharmacology of dimethyl sulfoxide in cardiac and CNS damage. Pharmacol Rep 2009;61(2):225–35.
29. Santos NC, Figueira-Coelho J, Martins-Silva J, et al. Multidisciplinary utilization of dimethyl sulfoxide: pharmacological, cellular, and molecular aspects. Biochem Pharmacol 2003;65(7):1035–41.
30. FDA/CVM. Food and Drug Administration Center for Veterinary Medicine final rule—extralabel drug use in animals. Fed Regist 1996;61:57731–46.
31. FDA/CVM. Animal drugs @ FDA, FDA approved animal drug products. 2014. Accessed October 26, 2014. Available at: http://www.accessdata.fda.gov/scripts/animaldrugsatfda/.

32. FDA. Food and drug administration grade "A" pasteurized milk ordinance. Food and Drug Administration. 2011. Accessed October 26, 2014. Available at: http://www.fda.gov/Food/GuidanceRegulation/GuidanceDocumentsRegulatory Information/Milk/ucm2007966.htm.
33. Cascino T, Baglivo J, Conti J, et al. Quantitative CT assessment of furosemide- and mannitol-induced changes in brain water content. Neurology 1983;33(7): 898–903.
34. Thenuwara K, Todd MM, Brian JE Jr. Effect of mannitol and furosemide on plasma osmolality and brain water. Anesthesiology 2002;96(2):416–21.
35. Todd MM, Cutkomp J, Brian JE. Influence of mannitol and furosemide, alone and in combination, on brain water content after fluid percussion injury. Anesthesiology 2006;105(6):1176–81.
36. Diringer MN, Zazulia AR. Osmotic therapy: fact and fiction. Neurocrit Care 2004; 1(2):219–33.
37. Candelise L, Colombo A, Spinnler H. Therapy against brain swelling in stroke patients. A retrospective clinical study on 227 patients. Stroke 1975;6:353–6.
38. Santambrogio S, Martinotti R, Sardella F, et al. Is there a real treatment for stroke? Clinical and Statistical comparison of different treatments in 300 patients. Stroke 1978;9:130–2.

Using Individual Animal Susceptibility Test Results in Bovine Practice

Brian Lubbers, DVM, PhD

KEYWORDS

- Antimicrobial susceptibility testing • AST • Veterinary diagnostic
- In vitro diagnostics • Responsible antimicrobial use

KEY POINTS

- Interpretive criteria developed by the Clinical and Laboratory Standards Institute for veterinary applications are specific to animal host species, bacterial pathogen, disease process, antimicrobial, and antimicrobial dosing regimen.
- Veterinary-specific interpretive criteria should be used (when available), because they provide the most predictive in vitro–in vivo relationship.
- When specific interpretive criteria do not exist for a veterinary application, laboratories may report interpretive criteria approved for other veterinary applications or developed from human data.
- When specific interpretive criteria do not exist for a veterinary application, practitioners can utilize specific microbiological, pharmacologic, and clinical evidence as an alternative to other veterinary or human breakpoints to evaluate antimicrobial therapies.

INTRODUCTION

Antimicrobial susceptibility testing (AST), as a laboratory procedure, was an integral part of the discovery of penicillin. In 1929, Alexander Fleming revolutionized modern medicine by describing a substance produced by *Penicillium,* which he termed "penicillin."[1] In that same article, Dr Fleming also described "Methods of examining cultures for antibacterial substance," an agar plate and broth dilution method, which are the precursors to modern AST. Shortly thereafter began the discussion on the utility of AST to predict clinical outcome,[2] a discussion that continues today.[3]

As testing methods have become standardized, AST reproducibility has been improved. To avoid many of the pitfalls AST can present, clinicians should verify

The author has nothing to disclose.
Kansas State Veterinary Diagnostic Laboratory, Kansas State University, 1800 Denison Avenue, Manhattan, KS 66506, USA
E-mail address: blubbers@vet.k-state.edu

Vet Clin Food Anim 31 (2015) 163–174
http://dx.doi.org/10.1016/j.cvfa.2014.11.008
0749-0720/15/$ – see front matter © 2015 Elsevier Inc. All rights reserved.

that their laboratory uses current testing methods and interpretive criteria approved by the Clinical and Laboratory Standards Institute (CLSI).[4]

Perhaps the most challenging aspect of AST lies in the interpretation and application of test results to the clinical patient. The value of cumulative AST data in empiric therapy for prescribing and monitoring of antimicrobial resistance has been discussed elsewhere.[5,6] The focus herein is on the application of AST results to the individual animal.

TERMINOLOGY

Although many of the technical aspects of how to perform AST in the laboratory have been standardized,[7,8] there remains a generalized lack of standardization of the terminology associated with this diagnostic test.[9] To fully comprehend AST results and their application to clinical case management, practitioners should understand the basic terminology associated with testing. For AST in North America, the primary entity that develops testing standards is CLSI. **Box 1** includes terms and definitions adapted from the most recent CLSI document.[10]

BREAKPOINT DEVELOPMENT PROCESS

A complete description of the process by which veterinary breakpoints are developed can be found in the most current CLSI document[11] and has been reviewed previously.[12,13] To develop a breakpoint, 3 types of data are used to determine the most appropriate cutoff values for "S," "I," and "R."

- Wild-type cutoff (CO_{wt}): The wild-type cutoff or minimum inhibitory concentration (MIC) distribution is a histogram of a population of bacterial isolates categorized by MIC value for an antibiotic (**Fig. 1**). The ultimate goal of the wild-type cutoff is to divide the bacterial population into 2 categories: wild type and non–wild type. Wild-type bacteria are ones that do not possess an acquired or mutational resistance element (ie, the susceptible population), whereas non–wild-type bacteria do possess these resistance characteristics. Because different bacterial species may have different MIC distributions to the same antimicrobial, breakpoint values are specific to an antimicrobial–bacterial pathogen combination.
- Pharmacokinetic/pharmacodynamics (PK/PD) cutoff ($CO_{pk/pd}$): The effectiveness of an antimicrobial agent is generally associated with 1 of 3 PK/PD indices: the time that free drug (non–protein bound) concentrations are greater than the MIC (f T>MIC), the free drug peak concentration to MIC ratio (f C_{max}:MIC), and the free drug area under the plasma concentration curve to MIC ratio (f AUC:MIC).[14] During the breakpoint development process, the pharmacokinetic properties of the specific antimicrobial in the host animal species are evaluated against the bacterial MICs to determine whether the target PK/PD index can be achieved. Because altering the dose regimen (increasing or decreasing the total dose or frequency of dosing, or using alternative routes of administration) will have an impact on the pharmacokinetic properties of the antimicrobial, breakpoint values are specific to the dose, route, and duration of therapy evaluated in the breakpoint development process. Many clinicians interpret this as meaning that a resistant isolate can be effectively treated by increasing the dose. This is not universally correct and this strategy should only be utilized in a few, specific clinical situations.
- Clinical cutoff (CO_{cl}): The final piece of data used to establish a veterinary breakpoint is to correlate in vivo treatment outcomes with the MIC of the specific

---

Box 1
Definitions

Broth (microwell) dilution testing

Antimicrobial susceptibility testing (AST) method that exposes the bacterial pathogen of interest to 2-fold dilutions of antimicrobial within a liquid culture media (broth). This is the most common test method used to determine the minimal inhibitory concentration.

Minimal Inhibitory Concentration (MIC)

The lowest concentration of an antimicrobial agent that prevents visible growth of a microorganism in a broth dilution susceptibility.

MIC_{50}/MIC_{90}

Values used to describe a population of bacterial isolates. Respectively, the MIC values at which 50% (MIC_{50}) and 90% (MIC_{90}) of the isolates in a population are at or below. For example, if 50% of the Mannheimia haemolytica isolates recovered from BRD submissions to a diagnostic laboratory had penicillin G MIC values at or below 0.5 μg/mL, the MIC_{50} would be 0.5 μg/mL **(Table 1)**. The MIC_{50} is not the concentration of antimicrobial that reduces growth within a single culture by 50%.

Disk diffusion testing

Test method that uses antimicrobial impregnated paper disks on a solid agar media to determine antimicrobial susceptibility of a bacterial pathogen. Also referred to as the Kirby–Bauer method.

Zone of inhibition

The measured zone around antimicrobial paper disks (for disk diffusion testing) where growth of bacteria was not observed.

Breakpoint/interpretive criteria

Minimal inhibitory concentration (MIC) or zone diameter value used to indicate susceptible ("S"), intermediate ("I"), or resistant ("R"). Throughout this article, the terms 'breakpoint' and 'interpretive criteria' are used interchangeably.

Susceptible

Category implies an infection that may be appropriately treated with the dosage regimen of an antimicrobial agent recommended for that type of infection and infecting (bacterial) species.

Intermediate

Category implies an infection that may be appropriately treated in body sites where the drugs are physiologically concentrated, or when a high dosage of drug can be used.

Resistant

Strains (in this category) are not inhibited by the usually achievable concentrations of the agent with normal dosage schedules and/or fall in the range (of MICs) where specific microbial resistance mechanisms are likely and clinical outcome has not been predictable in effectiveness studies.

---

bacterial pathogen causing disease. The clinical cutoff relationship is rarely straightforward, because it incorporates all of the "complicating" factors that relate to clinical outcome, such as host immune function and severity of the disease process. However, the general relationship will be that, as MIC values increase (bacteria demonstrate decreased susceptibility to the antimicrobial), clinical response decreases. The clinical cutoff is used to validate the preliminary breakpoint values determined from the wild-type and PK/PD cutoffs.

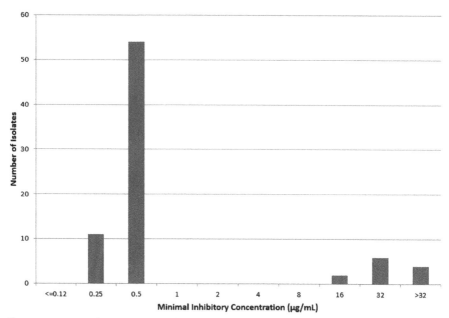

Fig. 1. Oxytetracycline minimum inhibitory concentration (MIC) distribution for *Mannheimia haemolytica* isolated from bovine respiratory disease submissions at Kansas State Veterinary Diagnostic Laboratory.

Currently, interpretive criteria for veterinary indications are established through a consensus process by the CLSI Veterinary Antimicrobial Susceptibility Testing subcommittee.[4] Breakpoints evaluated for an antimicrobial–bacterial pathogen–host species–disease process–dose regimen combination that have been formally developed by this committee using these 3 types of data are referred to as *veterinary-specific breakpoints*.

INTERPRETING TEST RESULTS WITH VETERINARY-SPECIFIC BREAKPOINTS

The relationship between AST and clinical outcome does not represent a perfect correlation.[15] Undoubtedly, most practitioners have experienced a case where the bacterial isolate was classified as "susceptible," and the patient failed to respond to therapy. In these cases, disease outcome may have been influenced by factors such as compromised host immune status, variation in individual host pharmacokinetics, and/or increased disease severity that could not be predicted by the in vitro antimicrobial–pathogen interaction.[16] What practitioners should expect is a reduction in clinical efficacy when a "resistant" bacterium is isolated. For this reason, when comparing 2 antimicrobials, both with veterinary-specific breakpoints, the prudent

Table 1
Penicillin G cumulative minimum inhibitory concentration (MIC) distribution for *Mannheimia haemolytica* isolated at Kansas State Veterinary Diagnostic Laboratory (n = 401)

MIC (µg/mL)	≤0.12	0.25	0.5[a]	1.0	2.0	4.0	8.0	≥16[b]
Isolates (cumulative), %	21	45	50	51	52	53	56	100

[a] MIC_{50} for the population of *Mannheimia haemolytica* isolates.
[b] MIC_{90} for the population of *Mannheimia haemolytica* isolates.

clinical decision is to select antimicrobials to which the given bacterium is "suscepti-ble" over the antimicrobial for which a "resistant" interpretation is given.

Of particular interest to the bovine practitioner, veterinary-specific breakpoints for cattle have only been developed for bovine respiratory disease (BRD) and mastitis. **Tables 2** and **3** list the antimicrobials and pathogens that have veterinary-specific interpretive criteria for these indications. When approved CLSI breakpoints are not available, laboratories may still report susceptibility testing results based on

Table 2
Antimicrobial–pathogen combinations with Clinical and Laboratory Standards Institute veterinary-specific breakpoints for bovine respiratory disease

Antimicrobial	Bacterial Pathogens
Ceftiofur	*Mannheimia haemolytica* *Pasteurella multocida* *Histophilus somni*
Danofloxacin[a]	*Mannheimia haemolytica* *Pasteurella multocida*
Enrofloxacin	*Mannheimia haemolytica* *Pasteurella multocida* *Histophilus somni*
Florfenicol	*Mannheimia haemolytica* *Pasteurella multocida* *Histophilus somni*
Gamithromycin[b]	*Mannheimia haemolytica* *Pasteurella multocida* *Histophilus somni*
Penicillin[c]	*Mannheimia haemolytica* *Pasteurella multocida* *Histophilus somni*
Spectinomycin	*Mannheimia haemolytica* *Pasteurella multocida* *Histophilus somni*
Tetracycline[d]	*Mannheimia haemolytica* *Pasteurella multocida* *Histophilus somni*
Tildipirosin[b]	*Mannheimia haemolytica* *Pasteurella multocida* *Histophilus somni*
Tilmicosin	*Mannheimia haemolytica*
Tulathromycin	*Mannheimia haemolytica* *Pasteurella multocida* *Histophilus somni*

[a] Only the susceptible breakpoint is established for this antimicrobial.
[b] Clinical and Laboratory Standards Institute–approved interpretive criteria are unpublished (CLSI, 2014) at this time, but can be obtained from the animal health company that markets the compound.
[c] Breakpoints apply only to the procaine penicillin G formulation used at 22,000 U/kg IM q24 h.
[d] Tetracycline is tested as the representative for this class of drug. Breakpoints apply only to paren-teral formulations (do not apply to feed medications).

Data from Clinical and Laboratory Standards Institute (CLSI). Performance standards for antimi-crobial disk and dilution susceptibility tests for bacteria isolated from animals; second informa-tional supplement. CLSI document VET01-S2. Wayne (PA): Clinical and Laboratory Standards Institute; 2013.

Table 3
Antimicrobial–pathogen combinations with Clinical and Laboratory Standards Institute veterinary-specific breakpoints for bovine mastitis

Antimicrobial	Bacterial Pathogens
Ceftiofur	*Staphylococcus aureus* *Streptococcus agalactiae* *Streptococcus dysgalactiae* *Streptococcus uberis* *Escherichia coli*
Penicillin (Novobiocin)	*Staphylococcus aureus* *Streptococcus agalactiae* *Streptococcus dysgalactiae* *Streptococcus uberis*
Pirlimycin	*Staphylococcus aureus* *Streptococcus agalactiae* *Streptococcus dysgalactiae* *Streptococcus uberis*

Data from Clinical and Laboratory Standards Institute (CLSI). Performance standards for antimicrobial disk and dilution susceptibility tests for bacteria isolated from animals; second informational supplement. CLSI document VET01-S2. Wayne (PA): Clinical and Laboratory Standards Institute; 2013.

interpretive criteria (S, I, R) for antimicrobial–pathogen combinations other than those listed in **Tables 2** and **3**; these interpretive criteria may be derived from other veterinary or human breakpoints, or possibly other sources and should be interpreted cautiously as a relationship between in vitro result–in vivo outcome may not exist.

BOVINE RESPIRATORY DISEASE

Applying AST results for cases of BRD is a relatively straightforward process, if the veterinarian is evaluating antimicrobials with veterinary-specific breakpoints. When comparing the antimicrobials listed in **Table 2**, AST results should be used to "rule out" antimicrobials to which the bacterial pathogen is "resistant." If the infecting pathogen is "susceptible" to multiple antimicrobials with veterinary-specific breakpoints, the practitioner should then use other factors (convenience of dosing, antimicrobial cost, tissue reactivity or others) to determine the most reasonable therapeutic option for that clinical situation. Again, it is not advised to compare antimicrobials with veterinary-specific breakpoints to antimicrobials with breakpoints derived from other sources (ie, other veterinary or human breakpoints) because the host-specific PK/PD, wild-type isolate distribution, and clinical outcome components are absent in the latter.

There are situations where clinicians may need to make relatively minor extrapolations to evaluate the utility of a specific antimicrobial. For example, tilmicosin BRD breakpoints exist only for *Mannheimia haemolytica*. If *Pasteurella multocida* is isolated from a specimen associated with clinical BRD, the clinician would preferentially select antimicrobials with veterinary breakpoints for *P multocida* over tilmicosin. However, if the situation exists where the antimicrobials with veterinary breakpoints are not valid therapeutic choices (ie, demonstrated lack of efficacy), the veterinarian can use the 3 types of data discussed (CO_{wt}, $CO_{pk/pd}$, CO_{cl}) to determine whether tilmicosin represents a reasonable treatment option.

Tilmicosin Wild-type Cutoff

If a MIC distribution is available to the practitioner (either through the practitioner's records or diagnostic laboratory summaries), an assessment of tilmicosin MICs for *P multocida* can be made. Ideally, there would be clear separation of wild-type (low MICs) and non–wild-type (high MICs) isolates. However, the example tilmicosin MIC distribution for *P multocida* isolates in **Fig. 2** does not clearly distinguish between wild-type and non–wild-type bacteria. There is a large group of *P multocida* isolates with MIC of 4 μg/mL or greater, with a trailing distribution of isolates at 8, 16, 32, 64, and 128 or greater μg/mL. Evaluation of the PK/PD relationship may provide more information in determining which MIC values represent a reasonable treatment option and which MIC values warrant considering another antimicrobial.

Tilmicosin Pharmacokinetic/pharmacodynamics Cutoff

The determination of a PK/PD response for bovine *P multocida* treated with tilmicosin would be a very complex process. Although pharmacokinetic data in cattle are available,[17] there is little information on the appropriate macrolide PK/PD index, location from which the pharmacokinetic data should be derived (ie, plasma, tissue, or pulmonary epithelial lining fluid), or magnitude of the pharmacodynamic index associated with antibiotic efficacy.[18] Rather, the clinician may assume (a very reasonable assumption in this author's opinion) that the pharmacokinetics of tilmicosin are similar in cattle affected with respiratory disease whether the pathogen is *M haemolytica* or *P multocida*. It is also reasonable to assume that the target pharmacodynamic index value would likely be unchanged between *M haemolytica* and *P multocida*. In **Fig. 3**, the interpretive criteria for *M haemolytica* have been inserted over the same tilmicosin MIC isolate distribution from **Fig. 2**. From this, the practitioner could infer that tilmicosin represents a reasonable therapeutic choice for *P multocida* isolates with MICs of less than 8 μg/mL (when other antimicrobials with veterinary-specific breakpoints are not valid options). These data suggest that tilmicosin is not a good therapeutic option for *P multocida* isolates with MICs of greater than 32 μg/mL.

Tilmicosin Clinical Cutoff

A true clinical cutoff is established by correlating pretreatment MIC values with the therapeutic outcome in an individual animal. Although this type of sampling is not

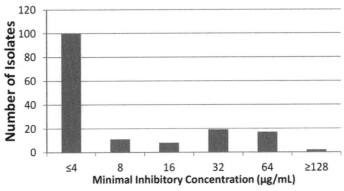

Fig. 2. Tilmicosin minimum inhibitory concentration distribution for *Pasteurella multocida* isolated from bovine respiratory disease submissions at Kansas State Veterinary Diagnostic Laboratory.

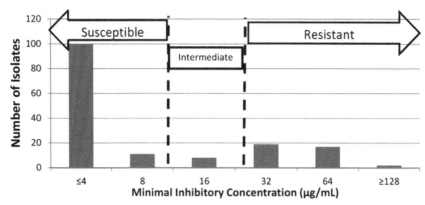

Fig. 3. Tilmicosin minimum inhibitory concentration distribution for *Pasteurella multocida* isolated from bovine respiratory disease submissions at Kansas State Veterinary Diagnostic Laboratory. The distribution shown is the same as for **Fig. 2** with an overlay of the interpretive criteria used for *Mannheimia haemolytica*.

common in daily practice, practitioners may be able to use ancillary evidence, such as treatment records and diagnostic reports, to further evaluate tilmicosin MICs for *P multocida*. Because the most common sample for BRD diagnostics is lung tissue from animals that have died from respiratory disease, this information is most likely to provide insight for *P multocida* isolates with higher MICs, that is, the MICs where tilmicosin should not be considered for therapy. For example, the use of *M haemolytica* tilmicosin breakpoints for *P multocida* is supported if *P multocida* isolates recovered from cattle that were treated with tilmicosin and died from BRD have MIC values of at least 32 μg/mL. Practitioners should avoid establishing a "clinical cutoff" based on a limited number of cases, because the multifactorial nature of BRD makes the correlation between MIC and clinical outcome imperfect at best.

INTERPRETING TEST RESULTS FOR OTHER DISEASE CONDITIONS

Pathogen–antimicrobial combinations for which there are no CLSI-approved veterinary breakpoints may also lack the standardized testing conditions that are necessary to ensure accurate test results.[19] However, in cases where no veterinary breakpoints exist for the specific disease in question, the practitioner can utilize the same types of evidence (CO_{wt}, $CO_{pk/pd}$, CO_{cl}) to evaluate whether a specific antibiotic is a reasonable or unreasonable therapeutic option. Using this approach may require the practitioner to make extrapolations within the data. However, in this context, the practitioner can use good professional judgment to ensure that the extrapolations being made are feasible and clinically reasonable. The interpretation of susceptibility testing for infectious bovine keratoconjunctivitis is a good example.

INFECTIOUS BOVINE KERATOCONJUNCTIVITIS (PINKEYE)

There are only 2 antimicrobials labeled for therapy of infectious bovine keratoconjunctivitis; injectable oxytetracycline (Liquamycin LA-200, Zoetis; Noromycin 300 LA, Norbrook; generic formulations) and tulathromycin (Draxxin, Zoetis). As such, the Animal Medicinal Drug Use Clarification Act[20] requires that veterinarians utilize one of these antimicrobials for treatment of this disease unless these antimicrobials have been shown to be ineffective clinically.

There are no CLSI-approved, veterinary-specific breakpoints for infectious bovine keratoconjunctivitis caused by *Moraxella bovis* or associated with *Moraxella bovoculi.* If susceptibility testing is being used as a guide for therapy in this situation, the practitioner could begin to determine the feasibility of either oxytetracycline or tulathromycin by obtaining MIC distributions from clinical case records, available published literature[21,22] or diagnostic laboratory summaries.

Evaluation of the *Moraxella* sp. MIC distribution for oxytetracycline (**Fig. 4**) shows a MIC distribution with most of the isolates testing at 0.5 μg/mL or less with a small number of isolates at 1, 2, 4, 8, and greater than 8 μg/mL. As in the previous example with *P multocida,* there is no clear distinction for where isolates become non–wild type (resistant).

Again, the practitioner could use PK/PD data to provide an assessment of reasonable MIC values for therapy with either oxytetracycline. Although the available literature provides some support for oxytetracycline concentrations in tear film,[23] only the use of free (non–protein-bound) *plasma* concentrations is considered appropriate for PK/PD.[24] Additionally, because the surface of the eye (tear film) is not an anatomically protected drug penetration site, the PK/PD component of other breakpoints in this species, BRD, for instance, would reasonably apply. In combination, these approaches would suggest that *Moraxella* isolates with MIC values of 0.5 or 1 μg/mL (the BRD susceptible breakpoint is ≤2 μg/mL) could be considered for treatment with parenteral oxytetracycline, whereas isolates with MIC values of greater than 8 μg/mL would warrant alternative antibiotic choices. For isolates with MIC values of 2 or 4 μg/mL, the practitioner may choose to consider alternative antibiotic therapies or use oxytetracycline at a higher dose (which would require extended withdrawal time). If the clinician chooses to use an extralabel dose of oxytetracycline for isolates with moderate MIC values (2, 4), treatment response rates should be monitored closely. The same approach could also be used to evaluate the utility of tulathromycin for infectious bovine keratoconjunctivitis therapy.

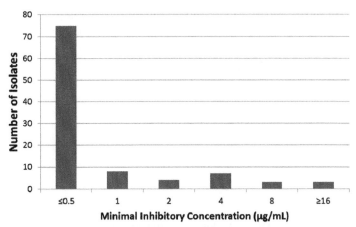

Fig. 4. Oxytetracycline minimum inhibitory concentration distribution for *Moraxella* spp. isolated from infectious bovine keratoconjunctivitis submissions at Kansas State Veterinary Diagnostic Laboratory. Distribution includes both *Moraxella bovis* and *Moraxella bovoculi* isolates.

SALMONELLOSIS

The initial consideration for the practitioner regarding salmonellosis is whether antimicrobial therapy is indicated or not. This decision will largely be based on the clinical presentation of the disease with aggressive supportive therapy (ie, fluids) being the mainstay of therapy for mild presentations of salmonellosis. There is evidence in the human medical literature that antimicrobial treatment of uncomplicated gastrointestinal disease can prolong the shedding of salmonella[25] and may increase the risk of disease relapse.[26] When indicated for human salmonellosis, fluoroquinolones are considered first-line antimicrobial therapy. Alternative first-line therapies include azithromycin, third-generation cephalosporins, trimethoprim–sulfamethoxazole, and ampicillin.[27]

Because there are no antimicrobials approved for treatment of *Salmonella* infections in cattle, any such use would be considered extralabel; thus, the fluoroquinolones would be excluded from consideration because there is a prohibition against extralabel use of this drug class in food animals. There are also no established susceptibility breakpoints for *Salmonella* sp. in cattle; any reported interpretive criteria will be adopted from other veterinary breakpoints, such as the BRD breakpoints in cattle, or from human susceptibility testing guidelines. The role of AST in a case such as this is to assist the practitioner in detecting *Salmonella* isolates with resistance elements and eliminating "unreasonable" therapeutic options.

As discussed for infectious bovine keratoconjunctivitis, the practitioner would begin with an evaluation of MIC distributions for *Salmonella.* For brevity, oxytetracycline is used as an example. The clinician would use the same process for any antimicrobial considered for therapy of *Salmonella* bacteremia.

As shown in **Fig. 5** for oxytetracycline, there are 2 populations of isolates. The isolates with MIC values of 16 μg/mL or greater would be classified as non–wild type and likely contain resistance genes that would result in decreased clinical efficacy of oxytetracycline.

Because the PK/PD component of oxytetracycline was evaluated in developing breakpoints for BRD ($\leq$2 μg/mL, susceptible; 4 μg/mL, intermediate; $\geq$8 μg/mL, resistant), these interpretive criteria could be evaluated against the wild-type distribution shown in **Fig. 5**. In doing so, it would be reasonable to extrapolate these breakpoints to *Salmonella* isolated from cattle. Isolates with MIC values of 8 μg/mL or greater should be considered resistant to oxytetracycline and the clinician should evaluate

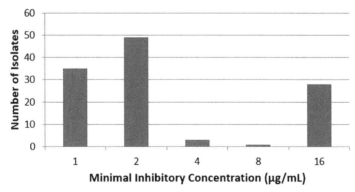

Fig. 5. Oxytetracycline minimum inhibitory concentration distribution for *Salmonella* spp. isolated from bovine submissions at Kansas State Veterinary Diagnostic Laboratory. Distribution includes all *Salmonella* species/serovars isolated from bovine cases.

alternative therapies. For "moderate" MIC values (4 μg/mL in this example), the clinician would either consider increasing the dose of oxytetracycline or selecting a different antimicrobial altogether, and oxytetracycline would be considered a reasonable therapeutic choice for isolates with MIC values of 2 μg/mL or less.

SUMMARY AND DISCUSSION

A significant amount of microbiological, pharmacologic, and clinical data is evaluated in establishing veterinary-specific interpretive criteria. The outcome of this process is an in vitro diagnostic test correlated with clinical efficacy (or lack of efficacy).[28] Owing to the inherent variability of biological systems and the multitude of factors that affect clinical outcome, this correlation is, and will continue to be, imperfect at best.[29] However, veterinary practitioners can fully realize the potential of this diagnostic test by (1) understanding whether the breakpoints being used are veterinary specific or have been adopted from other veterinary or human guidelines (or other sources); (2) preferentially using veterinary-specific breakpoints over breakpoints from other sources, when available; and (3), understanding which data extrapolations should and should not be made when veterinary-specific breakpoints do not exist.

When used in this manner, AST is a useful part of the antimicrobial selection process. Appropriately used, it can assist the veterinary practitioner in making, not only sound clinical judgments, but also ensures the most prudent use of antimicrobial agents.

REFERENCES

1. Fleming A. On the antibacterial action of cultures of a *Penicillium*, with special reference to their use in the isolation of *B. influenza*. Br J Exp Pathol 1929;10: 226–36.
2. Rodger KC, Branch A, Power EE, et al. Antibiotic therapy: correlation of clinical results with laboratory sensitivity tests. Can Med Assoc J 1956;74:605–12.
3. Greenwood D. In vitro veritas? Antimicrobial susceptibility tests and their clinical relevance. J Infect Dis 1981;144:380–5.
4. Schwarz S, Silley P, Simjee S, et al. Editorial: assessing the antimicrobial susceptibility of bacteria obtained from animals. J Antimicrob Chemother 2010;65:601–4.
5. El-Azizi M, Mushtaq A, Drake C, et al. Evaluating antibiograms to monitor drug resistance. Emerg Infect Dis 2005;11:1301–2.
6. Clinical and Laboratory Standards Institute (CLSI). Analysis and presentation of cumulative antimicrobial susceptibility test data; Approved guideline – 4th edition. CLSI document M39-A4. Wayne (PA): Clinical and Laboratory Standards Institute; 2014.
7. Bauer AW, Kirby WM, Sherris JC, et al. Antibiotic susceptibility testing by a standardized single disk method. Am J Clin Pathol 1966;45:493–6.
8. Clinical and Laboratory Standards Institute (CLSI). Performance standards for antimicrobial disk and dilution susceptibility tests for bacteria isolated from animals. CLSI document M31-A. Wayne (PA): Clinical and Laboratory Standards Institute; 1999.
9. Silley P. Susceptibility testing methods, resistance and breakpoints: what do these terms really mean? Rev Sci Tech 2012;31:33–41.
10. Clinical and Laboratory Standards Institute (CLSI). Performance standards for antimicrobial disk and dilution susceptibility tests for bacteria isolated from animals; approved standard – 4th edition. CLSI document VET01-A4. Wayne (PA): Clinical and Laboratory Standards Institute; 2013.

11. Clinical and Laboratory Standards Institute (CLSI). Development of in vitro susceptibility testing criteria and quality control parameters for veterinary antimicrobial agents; Approved guideline – 3rd edition. CLSI document VET02-A3. Wayne (PA): Clinical and Laboratory Standards Institute; 2008.

12. Watts JL, Yancey RJ. Identification of veterinary pathogens by use of commercial identification systems and new trends in antimicrobial susceptibility testing of veterinary pathogens. Clin Microbiol Rev 1994;7:346–56.

13. Jenkins SG, Jerris RC. Critical assessment of issues applicable to development of antimicrobial susceptibility testing breakpoints. J Clin Microbiol 2011;49:S5–10.

14. Ambrose PG, Bhavnani SM, Rubino CM, et al. Pharmacokinetics-pharmacodynamics of antimicrobial therapy: it's not just for mice anymore. Clin Infect Dis 2007;44:79–86.

15. Watts JL, Sweeney MT. Antimicrobial resistance in bovine respiratory disease pathogens: measures, trends, and impact on efficacy. Vet Clin North Am Food Anim Pract 2010;26:79–88.

16. Papich MG. Antimicrobials, susceptibility testing, and minimum inhibitory concentrations (MIC) in veterinary infection treatment. Vet Clin North Am Small Anim Pract 2013;43:1079–89.

17. Modric S, Webb AI, Derendorf H. Pharmacokinetics and pharmacodynamics of tilmicosin in sheep and cattle. J Vet Pharmacol Ther 1998;21:444–52.

18. Zhanel GG, Dueck M, Hoban DJ, et al. Review of macrolides and ketolides – focus on respiratory tract infections. Drugs 2001;61:443–98.

19. Apley MD. Susceptibility testing for bovine respiratory and enteric disease. Vet Clin North Am Food Anim Pract 2003;19:625–46.

20. CFR 530 extralabel drug use in animals - subpart C – specific provisions relating to extralabel use of animal and human drugs in food-producing animals. Available at: http://www.nrsp-7.org/Legislation/AMDUCA.pdf. Accessed August 7, 2014.

21. Angelos JA, Ball LM, Byrne BA. Minimum inhibitory concentrations of selected antimicrobial agents for *Moraxella bovoculi* associated with infectious bovine keratoconjunctivitis. J Vet Diagn Invest 2011;23:552–5.

22. Webber JJ, Fales WH, Selby LA. Antimicrobial susceptibility of *Moraxella bovis* determined by agar disk diffusion and broth microdilution. Antimicrob Agents Chemother 1982;21:554–7.

23. Punch PI, Costa ND, Chambers ED, et al. Plasma and tear concentrations of antibiotics administered parenterally to cattle. Res Vet Sci 1985;39:179–87.

24. Toutain PL, del Castillo JR, Bousquet-Mélou A. The pharmacokinetic-pharmacodynamic approach to a rational dosage regimen for antibiotics. Res Vet Sci 2002;73:105–14.

25. Aserkoff B, Bennett JV. Effect of antibiotic therapy in acute salmonellosis on the fecal excretion of Salmonellae. N Engl J Med 1969;281:636–40.

26. Nelson JD, Kusmiesz H, Jackson LH, et al. Treatment of *Salmonella* gastroenteritis with ampicillin, amoxicillin, or placebo. Pediatrics 1980;65:1125–30.

27. Sánchez-Vargas FM, Abu-El-Haija MA, Gómez-Duarte OG. *Salmonella* infections: an update on epidemiology, management, and prevention. Travel Med Infect Dis 2011;9:263–77.

28. Stratton CW. *In vitro* susceptibility versus *in vivo* effectiveness. Med Clin North Am 2006;90:1077–88.

29. Doern GV, Brecher SM. The clinical predictive value (or lack thereof) of the results of in vitro antimicrobial susceptibility tests. J Clin Microbiol 2001;49:S11–4.

Index

Note: Page numbers of article titles are in **boldface** type.

A

Acute interdigital necrobacillosis, **88–92**. *See also* acute interdigital necrobacillosis; foot rot; Infectious pododermatitis (IP)

α-2Adrenergic agonists
  in cattle, 130–131

Amoxicillin
  for mastitis in cattle, 22–27

Ampicillin
  for mastitis in cattle, 27

Analgesic(s)
  in cattle
    clinical pharmacology of, **113–138**. *See also specific drugs*
      introduction, 113–115
      local anesthesia, 116–120. *See also* Local anesthesia, in cattle, clinical pharmacology of
      neuropathic pain analgesics, 132
      NSAIDs, 120–129. *See also* Nonsteroidal anti-inflammatory drugs (NSAIDs), in cattle
      sedative-analgesic drugs, 129–132

Ancillary therapy
  in BRD management, 98

Anesthesia/anesthetics
  local
    in cattle
      clinical pharmacology of, 116–120. *See also* Local anesthesia, in cattle

Anti-inflammatory drugs
  for polioencephalomalacia in cattle, 155–158

Antibiotics
  in BRD management, 98–105
  in calf diarrhea management
    efficacy of, 52–53
    rationale for, 51–52
    types of, 53–56
  in calf diarrhea prevention, 49–51
  in mastitis management, 21–32. *See also specific drugs*
  in metritis management in dairy cattle, 140–145. *See also* Ceftiofur, in metritis management in dairy cattle

Antimicrobial decision making
  for enteric diseases of cattle, **47–60**. *See also* Enteric diseases, of cattle, antimicrobial decision making for

Antimicrobial drugs. *See* Antibiotics

http://dx.doi.org/10.1016/S0749-0720(15)00009-2
vetfood.theclinics.com

Moving?

Make sure your subscription moves with you!

To notify us of your new address, find your **Clinics Account Number** (located on your mailing label above your name), and contact customer service at:

Email: journalscustomerservice-usa@elsevier.com

800-654-2452 (subscribers in the U.S. & Canada)
314-447-8871 (subscribers outside of the U.S. & Canada)

Fax number: 314-447-8029

**Elsevier Health Sciences Division
Subscription Customer Service
3251 Riverport Lane
Maryland Heights, MO 63043**

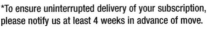

*To ensure uninterrupted delivery of your subscription, please notify us at least 4 weeks in advance of move.